ELEANOR T. CALVERLEY, M.D.

HOW TO BE HEALTHY IN HOT CLIMATES

SECOND EDITION

NEW YORK: THOMAS Y. CROWELL COMPANY

To my husband
EDWIN ELLIOTT CALVERLEY, Ph.D.

PREFACE

MANY INDIVIDUALS are being sent to the tropics on special missions. Such travelers are willing to accept any restrictions in order to return unscathed from countries where tropical diseases exist. It is for the needs of short-time travelers in an uncontrolled environment that maps, lists of diseases, a chart of precautions, and detailed information on immunizing procedures have been added in this edition (Appendix D).

The book was written originally for the author's missionary students. From her experience as a missionary physician and a mother in Arabia, she wished to make available something which she had been unable to find: a handbook for lay persons on the subjects of tropical hygiene and tropical diseases. Long-time residents in the tropics, such as these students in Hartford, Connecticut, at the Kennedy School of Missions of the Hartford Seminary Foundation, face a situation which is different from that of the short-time traveler. While planning to make the controlled environment of their homes as safe as possible for themselves and their families, readers of this sort are aware that a certain amount of risk to their health, through the acceptance of hospitality and the performance of their duties, is inherent in their vocation. They see many of their predecessors who have lived successfully and brought up their families without casualties in the countries where they intend to live. And they can hope that through necessary exposure to infection through the years, a degree of immunity or tolerance to disease germs may be acquired.

In the first printing of this book acknowledgment was made of assistance received from many friends, medical and otherwise. To the list of valued advisers new names are now added. These include Dr. Harold N. Mozar, Director of the School of Tropical and Preventive Medicine of the College of Medical Evangelists, Loma Linda, California. Our debt is acknowledged also to Dr. Dewey Katz, a leading ophthalmologist of Hartford, Connecticut, for help in bringing up to date the chapter on diseases of the eye.

Through the continued interest of Dr. Hazel M. Hauck, Professor of Food and Nutrition of the New York State College of Home Economics, at Cornell University, the help of a trained nutritionist, Mary Katharine Russell, M.S., was enlisted for revising chapter 10 and Appendix A on the subject of food. Miss Russell has taught nutrition both in the United States and at Cheeloo University and Ginling College in China. Her table of food values in Appendix A, featuring especially foods available in the tropics, is considered by the author to be one of the outstanding improvements offered in this edition.

CONTENTS

▀▀

v

IS IT SAFE TO LIVE IN THE TROPICS?

"YOU'LL MAKE a good meal for some cannibal!" The remark was made in fun to a young doctor preparing for service in Arabia, but it well illustrates the vague fears with which most of us regard the tropics, a region of extreme heat and mysterious, deadly diseases.

If you intend to go to a hot country, how can you reassure yourself and your friends as to your relative safety and comfort? Will it be safe to live in such a climate? What precautions can you take, and against what? The answer to these questions must depend on several considerations. First, where exactly are you going? What sort of person are you, and what preparation will you have for the life in such a place?

Where Are You Going?

It is quite possible that you may receive an agreeable surprise. The regions generally known as "the tropics" vary greatly in respect to climate, living conditions, and potential disease hazards. Moreover, some sections may prove particularly dangerous to some people, while others may live there in relative safety.

Climate. The words *tropics* and *tropical* will be used in this book in a broad sense as denoting places in hot parts of the world, irrespective of latitude or average annual temperature.

One of the circumstances affecting climate is altitude. In India, for example, a few hours travel can take one from the intense heat of the lowlands to the delightful coolness of snow-covered mountains. Even at sea level and with equal degrees of temperature, climates vary greatly in respect to humidity. A temperature of 90 degrees [1] where the air is moist may be much more uncomfortable than a far higher temperature where the air is dry.

Prevailing winds are another modifying factor. A cool breeze from the sea can make life quite pleasant in some hot parts of the world, but where mountains shut off all cooling air currents, the average Westerner is compelled to go away on vacation during the worst months. In other places, there may be times when a scorching wind blowing over the desert burns up the countryside.

It is unlikely that the foreigner will be expected to live in a trying climate without the respite of an occasional holiday. But if the prospective traveler has any misgivings about his ability to adjust to whatever climatic conditions he may meet, he should make inquiry about the specific circumstances in the place he expects to visit.

Living Conditions. In a metropolis such as Bombay or Cairo, the chances are that you will live in a modern apartment with most of the conveniences. Your way of life in such a case may be very similar to what it has been at home.

Even in places remote from the city, you can have pleasant living quarters. Refrigeration, air conditioning, radio, and air transportation have made a great difference in tropical living. Some adjustment must be made however, no matter how favorable the situation. And only those with a high degree of adaptability and much resourcefulness should be sent to the more difficult stations, where there may be appreciable deprivations.

Potential Disease Hazards. Many foreigners experience no ill effects from living in hot countries. The first five years are the decisive period. If one remains in good health during these years, he may well be given a preferred insurance rating.

Statistics are needed in order to evaluate potential hazards

[1] Temperatures given refer to the Fahrenheit scale unless otherwise indicated.

in any particular location. Dr. Wm. G. Lennox' *The Health and Turnover of Missionaries* [2] contains graphs and information indicating proportionate causes of death and invaliding illnesses occurring in those parts of the world that we have in mind.

Degenerative Conditions. It will be seen from these graphs that the largest number of deaths and the next to largest number of withdrawals are due to degenerative conditions including some diseases of the heart, the blood vessels, the kidneys, and the like. Such diseases are likely to occur with advancing years in any place, but in hot countries the process of degeneration may have been speeded by an unfavorable environment.

Common Infections. Next to degenerative disease as a cause of death and fourth in the graph of invaliding illnesses are the common infections, which occur frequently outside the tropics.

Tropical Infections. The third section in both graphs is allotted to tropical infections. Although these constitute the class of hazards most closely associated with tropical countries, some of them occur in the temperate zones. It should be remembered, too, that this record covers a period when many of today's facilities for immunization and for treatment of disease were unknown.

Today, we can be vaccinated against a number of tropical infections. The use of DDT as an insecticide, which appreciably cut down infestations and illness in the armed forces during World War II, should do much to maintain health in the future. New drugs are now available for treatment and air travel should to an increasing degree make it possible to secure medical and surgical care quickly, even for those who live far from hospitals and doctors.

A few *rules for safety* need to be learned by the traveler before he starts his journey. By avoiding unsafe food and drink (see Appendix D, IV) he will usually be protected against the dysenteries—amoebic and bacillary. These are so common that no map has been prepared to depict their incidence. Other intestinal infections are prevented by the same precau-

[2] Methodist Book Concern, New York.

tions. To protect against malaria, in regions shown on the map to be malarious (Appendix D), one must sleep under a bed net. This measure, together with the use of a repellent, DDT powder, and an aerosol bomb, should protect against other insect-borne diseases. In regions where the snail-borne disease schistosomiasis ("fluke" disease) is found (see map in Appendix D), contact of the skin with untreated water (page 214), as in wading or bathing, must be avoided. To protect against hookworm disease, widespread in tropical and semi-tropical regions, one should not walk barefoot on the soil. A summary of precautions to be followed in tropical areas will be found in Appendix D, IV.

Functional Nervous Disorders. In Dr. Lennox' report 29 per cent of the invaliding conditions fall into the category commonly known as "nerves." Many individuals are unsuited for any situation involving unusual strain and stress. In the selection of workers for tropical countries, careful consideration should be given to the individual's emotional and nervous stability.

What Sort of a Person Are You?

Southern and eastern countries are full of color and charm. Can you enjoy them? Have you noticed people on furlough from the tropics—how eager they are to get back? In many ways life in hot parts of the world is more enjoyable than in the temperate zones. Does the prospect of a life totally different from what you've known give you a feeling of adventure? But can you, if necessary, do without luxuries and "rough it"?

Can you associate in a friendly way with all kinds of people, regardless of culture or race? Are you overdominant or bossy—or afflicted with self pity? Have you any strongly marked fears of anything—insects or germs, for instance. Can you be depended on to take sane and practical measures about such things, instead of wasting nervous energy in fear? Can you bear sights that shock the senses?

Are you genuinely interested in your work? Have you at least one hobby, as a safeguard against boredom? How have

you reacted *in the past* to upsetting situations? When the sled-
ding was rough, could you take it?

Have you been able to get along with people in the past? To
be associated constantly and intimately with an uncongenial
person is always unpleasant, but in a lonely station, with few
resources for diversion, petty difficulties assume large proportions. Patience, tolerance, tact, and a very real *desire to like*
an associate is vitally necessary in order to live beside a person
whose temperament is incompatible with one's own.

Can you keep your temper? To the Oriental mind a lack of
self-control is one of the worst of faults. Perfection, of course,
is out of the question. A sense of humor, however, can be a
wonderfully redeeming trait. During a time of unusual danger
in an Eastern city, when everyone's nerves were at the breaking
point, someone introduced a rhyme about:

> The cow's in the hammock!
> The baby's in the lake!
> The cat's in the garbage!—
> What difference does it make?

The nonchalant absurdity of that summary of disasters drew
a roar of laughter from the worried little group, and broke up
the tension completely.

2

PREPARATION FOR LIFE IN THE TROPICS

JUST AS special qualifications are needed for life in the tropics, so special preparations are obviously desirable. The first of these should be a thorough physical examination. After this, provided acceptance of the applicant is assured, three further measures should be taken. These are: health service, including correction of defects and abnormalities discovered by the doctor; immunization against certain diseases; and education in tropical hygiene.

The Health Examination

Most organizations provide the applicant for tropical service with a printed form on which results of the physical examination are to be recorded by the physician. This schedule begins with questions about age and weight. The immature are at a disadvantage under circumstances demanding unusual physical stamina. Women under twenty-one especially are said to have low resistance to heat and humidity. Persons over forty, also, may find it difficult to make adjustment to the tropics. The overweight and the undernourished also are less well adapted for enduring hot climates.

While the doctor's examination will be made with care, there are certain minor disabilities which can best be determined by the individual himself. A good digestion is particularly important. Those with sluggish livers, irritable colons, or a history of gall-bladder disease which may recur, are unlikely to thrive in the tropics.

Undiscovered tubercular infection is likely to flare up after one has reached the tropics. If there is any uncertainty on this point, an X-ray study of the chest is advisable. Sinus trouble, asthma, and chronic bronchitis are likely to become more troublesome in warm and humid climates.

Health Service—Correction of Abnormalities

Any physical defect which may cause trouble later should be corrected, if possible, before one goes to the tropics. Operations for such conditions as diseased tonsils, hemorrhoids (piles), chronic appendicitis, or hernia (rupture) should not be put off. Trusses for control of hernia are not satisfactory for use in hot climates.

A complete dental survey should be made and the teeth should be in as nearly perfect condition as possible. When dentures are needed, the provision of duplicates is a wise precaution to insure against breakage. For those who wear glasses, it is a good idea to take along at least two pairs. In any event, a copy of the prescription for glasses should be retained for future reference.

Special Service for Women. Women, married or single, should receive a thorough pelvic examination. Menstrual difficulties or other related handicaps ought to receive careful attention. A warm climate may have a beneficial effect on periodic pain due to spasm but, on the other hand, excessive bleeding is likely to increase under these circumstances. When the latter condition is due to tumor, however slight, rapid growth is likely to occur after one reaches the tropics, and serious hemorrhage may begin at a time when surgical assistance is not available. Much of this trouble can be avoided at the outset by a simple operation.

Immunization Against Disease

Before beginning his journey, the individual may receive a series of injections to make him immune to some of the most dangerous diseases to which he may be exposed. In rare cases where a disease is contracted despite such preventive measures, symptoms are usually mild, and the illness is not severe. Most governments require the International Certificate of Vaccination signed by the doctor at the time of immunization and certified afterward in regard to smallpox and cholera vaccination by a health officer. Information as to what immunizations are required by the particular country or countries to be visited or passed through at the time of your travel are summarized in Appendix D, III. They are given in detail in the current issue of the pamphlet *Immunization Information for International Travel,* obtainable from Federal Security Agency, Public Health Service, Washington 25, D.C. (at the price of 20 cents). International Certificates, usually sent to the traveler by the Department of State after application has been made for a passport, or furnished by travel agencies, can be purchased at the price of 5 cents from the Superintendent of Documents, U.S. Government Printing Office, Washington 25, D.C.

Basic Plan for Immunization

Usually all immunizations except for yellow fever (required at present for most of Africa and South America and for Republic of Panama, including the Canal Zone) can be performed by your own physician. Yellow fever inoculations are given at specified stations of the United States Public Health Service. Information not supplied by your sponsoring agency may be secured from the Office of International Relations, Public Health Service, Washington 25, D.C.

Certain countries (see page 276) require, in addition to the International Certificate of Vaccination, a health certificate from a doctor stating that the traveler is in good physical and mental health.

The traveler may wish to keep for his own future reference a record of immunizations given before travel.

It is well when possible, to have immunization finished three weeks before the date of expected departure. The normal interval between the first and last injection is six weeks, so an appointment with the doctor must not be put off until the last minute. In emergencies when a traveler must leave on short notice certain injections can be combined and the last ones given en route.

Most of us suffer little real inconvenience from immunization. The first and second doses of typhoid-paratyphoid vaccine are the two most likely to cause chills, fever, and headache. Even these cause some people no discomfort other than a red and swollen arm which is not truly painful.

It is taken for granted that children will have had the usual immunization given to babies. In the tropics vaccination against smallpox must be given very early, sometimes as early as the tenth day of life and repeated if necessary, monthly, until a "take" is secured. Thousands of native babies are killed or blinded by smallpox.

Repeat and Booster Vaccinations. Permanent protection against any disease cannot be expected. In some places it is thought wise to vaccinate against smallpox every year. The complete course of typhoid-paratyphoid vaccine may be given every two years; or one injection yearly may be preferred by your doctor. At times of unusual danger, as in case of an epidemic, an extra "booster" dose of any immunizing agent may be needed. Or at the time of a wound thought to be susceptible to tetanus infection, the doctor may give a booster shot of tetanus toxoid.

Education in Tropical Hygiene

The principal dangers for which the traveler must be prepared are the dysenteric diseases and malaria. There is no vaccination against these infections. The individual must protect himself by his own carefulness in avoiding sources of infection. Circumstances vary greatly. There are travelers who are fully protected by first class transportation agencies until they reach their destination. Others will be subjected to the danger of using unsafe drinking water and food and of being bitten by malarial mosquitoes. They must know the dangers and how to avoid them and they must have the strength of purpose to use the precautions which they know.

A course in tropical hygiene should be a great help to a

person intending to go to the tropics. But, reduced to their lowest terms, needed precautions are very simple. A person reading page 3 and following those instructions carefully would be safer than one who has studied extensively and fails to put into practice the knowledge he gains. Precautions soon become habitual and are taken in one's stride without worry or concern.

There is nothing in the mere crossing of an ocean to make a careless person careful. Begin *now,* even where special precautions are not needed, to work and play, eat, sleep and exercise as you know you should. And train yourself *now* in sane habits and healthy thinking about your body.

3

EQUIPMENT FOR THE TRAVELER

Passport and Travelers' Checks

Application for your passport should be made some months in advance of the anticipated date of departure. Apply for visas from the consular authorities of each of the countries that you may visit en route. Such visas are required for going ashore while in port in any country, even though one does not make a stop between ships or travel through it.

Travelers' checks are the safest and most convenient way to carry money. Check numbers should be noted and carried separately from the checks, in case of loss or theft. The loss of passport, travelers' checks, or money is a serious matter. While on shipboard, leave these with the purser. At all other times carry them in a pocket that is securely fastened.

How to Plan

Selection and packing of supplies is a matter that varies according to circumstances. Advice should be sought from persons acquainted with the place to which you are going. For the actual voyage, luggage such as suitcases, steamer trunk, and canvas duffel bag may be kept in the cabin. Larger trunks and packing cases are stored in the ship's hold. House furnishings and such are usually packed in boxes and sent off by freight months in advance of the passenger.

Planning for Enjoyment and Comfort. You will need books, newspapers, and magazines. They may have to take the place of lectures, conferences, conversation, and other means of keeping up-to-date. Subscribe to as many publications as you can afford, particularly those dealing with your work or hobbies. Don't neglect periodicals in the lighter vein; they can be as important to you as the serious. Persons who have children should keep them in mind, too, when considering a choice of reading matter.

For those who love music a phonograph is a priceless possession. Records packed carefully, with plenty of corrugated paper for padding, can be shipped without breakage. And don't forget a supply of phonograph needles.

Electrical Equipment.[1] Before you pack your electrical appliances, determine whether electric current is available in the region where you are to live. If so, is the current direct or alternating, what voltage and frequency? Most equipment manufactured for use in the United States is for 110-volt, 60-cycle frequency. In foreign countries this current is very often not found.

In many devices the voltage for alternating current can be adjusted by a transformer. Let an electrician advise you on this point; tell him what current is available and what devices you wish to use. In the matter of radios, it is better to consult the manufacturer rather than a dealer. The factory can supply an attachment which will give good performance; many dealers are unfamiliar with the problem, since it never arises in the States.

It is wise to consult a dealer as to whether it is more practical to change or adapt the equipment to the available current or to install a transformer. He will need the following information about the current in use at your destination:

> Is current direct or alternating?
> What is the voltage?
> What is the cycle?
> What is the phase?

[1] For the following information we are indebted to Professor H. W. Vandersall, Professor of Physics at the American University at Cairo, Egypt.

Household Needs. Take several cookbooks. A refrigerator is a necessity; and, if electricity is unavailable, a kerosene-operated refrigerator may be used. Other helpful appliances are a deep freeze, an air conditioner, a dehumidifier, and a pressure cooker.

Oil heaters, during a cold or rainy season, are a genuine comfort. Although your cook may use wood or charcoal as fuel, an oil stove with an oven will be an inestimable convenience. A generous supply of wicks and replacements for parts that may wear out should be provided, too.

A meat grinder is essential in places where meat is nearly always tough. It is also a good idea to take along a half dozen of such perishable and inexpensive items as strainers and egg beaters.

Packing

Companies specializing in exporting to foreign countries are equipped to pack efficiently, but even these should be cautioned to use more than the usual care with goods to be shipped to the tropics. Any goods which are to be packed by the individual himself should be boxed with great care. As a rule small boxes are preferable to larger and more cumbersome ones. Fastening them with screws will facilitate customs inspections. Hinges and padlocks may be used on covers, but padlocks are sometimes broken off during the journey. Boxes should be lined with waterproof material, such as tarred paper or oilcloth.

For your own use you will wish to have a list of the contents of each box. On the other hand, for the purpose of customs declaration, all articles of the same sort should be listed together (glass and crockery, household linen, etc.) regardless of the container. The approximate value of each group should be stated. Make a point of inquiring about the customs regulations in the particular country to which you are going.

Wearing Apparel

Warm Clothing. Provision should be made for cold days, even in the tropics. At one stage or another, the traveler is likely to feel the need for a warm coat, a sweater, or even a steamer rug. A waterproof coat with a detachable warm lining will serve for all kinds of weather.

For the journey, nylon garments of all types, which can be washed out over night, are a great convenience.

Cool Clothing. Perspiration in the tropics necessitates frequent changes of outer garments as well as underwear. All of these should be of the thinnest, most porous material available. Light colors are coolest and white has the advantage of absorbing the least heat.

Dresses for women in the tropics call for lines that will look well without tight foundation garments. However, few articles of one's wardrobe need be left behind. There are times when almost any type of clothing will be useful.

Formal Dress. Pack at least one formal evening costume where it will be available during the voyage. It is customary to dress for the "Captain's dinner" on the last night of an ocean voyage. At your destination, too, however out-of-the-way it may be, evening clothes may be socially essential. Extreme décolletage is unsuitable, especially in those countries where it is the custom for women of the country to veil their faces.

Sunglasses, Hats, Topees, and Umbrellas. Sunglasses should always be available. Perhaps at some tropical port en route you will feel the need for a topee or sun helmet as a protection against the sun. It is better to wait and buy one of the particular style in favor at your place of destination, except in cases of real need. Wearing an ordinary hat and carrying an umbrella, when the heat is intense, is usually sufficient.

Shoes. Shoes present a major problem for those who live in distant places. An adequate supply of footwear for all kinds of weather and for all occasions is eminently desirable. Those with entirely normal feet may adapt themselves to the foreign make of shoes, but many residents find it desirable to make arrangements with a good shoe store to keep a record of the size and kind of shoe they need, so that supplies can be ordered at intervals.

White shoes, of canvas or linen, are coolest. Rubber soles are not advised. Sizes for hot weather should allow for a little swelling of the feet, owing to the heat. Some women report needing two sizes larger than usual. With suits, coats, and dresses, the opposite is true—they are better made to fit snugly, or they will be too loose after the warm climate has had its usual "slimming" effect.

Needs for Air Travel

The luggage to be carried by an air traveler is usually restricted to forty or fifty pounds. It takes careful planning to include in this allowance clothing for all kinds of weather. Garments worn while embarking are not included in the baggage weighed. One can wear a waterproof coat with a detachable woolen lining over a suit. It is sometimes very cold at high altitudes and a steamer rug carried on the arm or strapped to the suitcase will be useful. In your pockets you may carry various articles, such as a little cotton or tissue to protect the ear drums from sudden change in atmospheric pressure. A "pocket toilet kit" containing soap, a wash cloth, and some toilet tissue is recommended. Washrooms along the way often contain neither soap, towels nor tissue. A small flashlight will come in handy when washrooms are dark.

Needs en Route

Whether one travels by sea, land, or air one may need Dramamine for motion sickness (page 17). Those who travel all the way under expert supervision may not need to provide a "mosquito bar," insecticides, or tablets for making water safe to drink. Others who may spend nights in hotels in malarious regions may find bed nets there nonexistent or in poor repair. And some ships as well as hotels come equipped with bedbugs. If one has provided a bed net, DDT powder, an aerosol bomb, and a repellent (see page 263), he is prepared to deal with any insects. And a supply of Globaline tablets (Wallace and Tiernan, Belleville 9, N.J.) will make dubious water safe for drinking.

Your First Aid Kit

This is required equipment. For average travelers a small tin box, such as is sold commercially, will serve the purpose. It should contain the following: (1) a small bottle of antiseptic (mercurochrome is usual, but tincture of Zephiran or 2% tincture of iodine is better); (2) aromatic spirits of ammonia, in bottle or ampules; (3) a tube of burn ointment; (4) compact supplies of sterile cotton, bandages, individual dressings with adhesive plaster, and a few sterile gauze compresses; and (5) a small roll of adhesive tape and a pair of scissors.

Desirable additions to the kit will be suggested by the reading of Appendix C. One should certainly have a clinical thermometer or two, together with a mild laxative, aspirin, and soda mints or Creamalin tablets for indigestion. Allergic persons will need to take tablets such as pyribenzamine. Where there are children, castor oil is likely to be needed (page 184) and syrup of ipecac for croup. For time of illness, parents should provide food such as Cream of Wheat, powdered milk or Mul Soy, and easily digested crackers—articles which are not always available on ships. Vaseline, boric acid (in powder form or tablets) to use as eye drops and for other purposes, and a combined hot water bottle and fountain syringe may prove very useful.

Travelers who may be for considerable periods without medical supervision in places where malaria and the dysenteries are common should provide themselves with remedies for these diseases. Aralen, milibis, and terramycin, are suggested. Two weeks before reaching a malarious region one should begin taking suppressive treatment with aralen, as outlined on page 141. For *short* stays where amoebic dysentery is prevalent, milibis may be used in *prevention* of that disease. An adult or child weighing over 80 pounds may be given one tablet containing 0.5 gm. three times a day for seven days. Children weighing less than 80 pounds should be given half this dose. Tablets containing 0.25 gm. are available. Tablets are also available combining milibis (0.25 gm.) with aralen (75.0 mg.) for killing amoeba inside the intestine and elsewhere in the body.

Each traveler must get as much information as possible about the journey and the places he is to visit. He can then choose his equipment with intelligence.

orrection for *How to Be Healthy in Hot Climates*
by Eleanor T. Calverley

age 16, line 15 from bottom through line 4 from
bottom should read: for these diseases.
Aralen is suggested for malaria (page
147), sulfadiazine for bacillary dysentery
(page 182), and tablets of milibis with
aralen for amoebic dysentery. For
treatment of amoebic dysentery in a person
weighing over 80 pounds, the dose of
milibis with aralen is two tablets three
times a day for seven days. For those
weighing less than eighty pounds half this
dose is to be given.

Two weeks before reaching a highly
malarious region one should begin taking
suppressive treatment of malaria with
aralen as outlined on page 141. For
short stays in places where amoebic
dysentery is very prevalent and sanitation
poor, milibis with aralen may be used in
prevention of that disease. The adult
dose for *prevention* is two tablets as a
single dose daily for not more than three
months. On page 279 reference will be
found to the use of diodoquin tablets for
a period of 20 days in prevention of
amoebic dysentery. The dosage of diodoquin
for *both treatment and prevention* is as
follows: for an adult or a child weighing
over 30 pounds one tablet containing 0.650
gm. is to be taken three times a day for
20 days. For children weighing less than
30 pounds the dose is half a tablet. The
use of sulfadiazine in prevention of
bacillary dysentery is explained on page
182.

Refreshments upon Landing. Upon landing from a plane or a ship, one's first move is probably to get refreshments. But be very careful what you drink. Do not drink the local water. Hot tea and coffee are usually safe. Evaporated milk, straight from the can may be used; but fresh milk and milk products or canned milk diluted with water must be avoided. Ice cream is not safe to eat. And in any hot climate the danger of eating custard type of foods, like cream puffs, in which germs multiply quickly in the absence of careful refrigeration, is well known. Pastries and sweets which have been exposed to flies are also dangerous. But cookies and sweets fresh from tin cans may be enjoyed.

In restaurants choose hot, well-cooked foods and hot drinks. Especially avoid salads because of the likelihood that such foods have had contact with fertilizer containing human excreta. These often contain germs of dysentery, typhoid fever, intestinal worms, or cholera.

Fruits with thick skins, like oranges and bananas may be considered safe after careful washing and scalding and removal of the skin. Fruits are often freshened in a ditch or puddle before marketing. Melons are sometimes pricked full of holes and soaked in unsafe water to increase their weight. No amount of washing would make these safe.

Apart from the foregoing, bottled drinks of known make and unbroken seal may be trusted. Otherwise bottles may have been refilled with unsafe beverages. Open the bottle yourself and allow no contact of the beverage with ice, which may have been made from unsafe water.

Wash your hands before eating. In places where intestinal diseases are common, disease-producing organisms are likely to be on almost anything you touch. Form the habit of washing your hands frequently, and keep your hands away from the mouth or eyes. But avoid going to ridiculous extremes in these practices.

Germs vs. Worry. Don't develop a phobia about germs. One anxious housewife asked what disinfectant she should use for washing dishes in her new Middle Eastern home! The usual soap and hot water are quite adequate for this purpose except in special cases of illness. Another timid individual, invalided home largely because of emotional instability, refused to take his books with him, fearing they might have been contaminated by contact with polluted air.

There are times when you may have to take a chance with germs. In such a case, do not frighten yourself into a state of panic. Someone has described worry as "a circle of inefficient thinking whirling about an axis of fear." This state of mind sometimes does more harm than bacteria. It never helps.

The majority of travelers make the journey to their destination under competent supervision. Extra money spent for transportation and hotel accommodations through dependable agencies is not wasted. Cut-rate companies may have poorly trained cooks and inadequate refrigeration of food. Luxury is not essential; precaution against disease is.

SUGGESTED READING

Victor Heiser, M.D., *An American Doctor's Odyssey*, W. W. Norton & Company, Inc., New York, 1936.

George K. Strode, M.D., et al., *Health Hints for the Tropics* (23 pages), Supplement to *Tropical Medicine and Hygiene News*, published by The American Society of Tropical Medicine and Hygiene with the sponsorship of the American Foundation for Tropical Medicine. Copies may be obtained from the American Foundation for Tropical Medicine, 345 Madison Ave., New York 17, N.Y., at 25 cents per copy. Quantities may be had at reduced rates.

5

ADJUSTING TO THE NEW ENVIRONMENT

▀▀▀

UPON ARRIVAL at one's destination, one finds his future friends and associates living normally and successfully in this unaccustomed place. He finds that these people go about their work and recreation with easy friendliness, despite the intense warmth which seems to him so uncomfortable. How is it that they do not break down, give up the job which brought them to this place?

One answer is that they have learned to emulate the nationals of the country in their daily routine. Although these residents rise at the first hint of dawn, they live at a more leisurely pace than is customary in cooler climates. At noon the shops and offices are closed for several hours. It is the time for lunch and a siesta.

As an example of the routine that one may expect, the following is typical of the life of an English household in India. Awakened early by a manservant bringing in a tray, one is served a breakfast—tea, toast with butter and marmalade, fresh fruit. This is the "chota hazri," or little breakfast. When one has bathed and dressed, this cooler part of the morning is devoted to the more strenuous part of his exercise and work. A few hours later, breakfast is served, a hearty meal beginning with porridge as a rule. Then work is resumed.

At one or two o'clock, lunch, or tiffin, is served. After this meal, most people retire for an hour or more of rest before returning to work. The next pause in the day's work is at four or five o'clock, when afternoon tea is taken. This is the hour for receiving guests and relaxing in an atmosphere of pleasant hospitality.

Very busy people may have to return to work, but as the day grows cooler many go out for a ride through the country-side or play tennis or badminton. Then, after a shower and change of clothes, one is ready for dinner at around eight o'clock. Earlier it is usually too warm for enjoyment of the evening meal. The remainder of the evening is given over to entertainment and recreation.

Wherever you may go in the tropics you will find such a schedule, with minor modifications. It is unwise to reject customs and practices which have evolved through years of experience. Those zealous persons who take no time off for relaxation, exercise, and sociability are making a grave mistake.

Hygiene in the Tropics

Food and Drink. Care in avoiding unsafe food and drink should soon be an automatic thing. The desirability of a balanced diet is obvious. But the homemaker will be faced with another problem. Continued hot weather is likely to result in loss of appetite. Much can be done to avoid this by making the home, and the dining room in particular, as cool and attractive as possible. In a hot, dry climate, the house should be closed and darkened against the heat while the air is still cool in the morning. The relief of coming into a relatively cool and shaded dwelling after the hot glare of midday is keenly appreciated.

A daintily set table and a delicious meal, well-balanced and appetizing, accompanied by cheerful conversation favor the survival of a good appetite in hot weather. Highly spiced dishes are favorites in hot countries and, taken in moderation, are a useful addition to the diet. Served too frequently, they may stimulate a tendency to overeat and to indulge to excess in alcoholic beverages. Such overindulgence may lead to a condition known as tropical liver, changing a normal, pleasant person into a jaundiced, ill-tempered dyspeptic.

Although constipation may be a problem for some people in warm climates, the opposite condition of diarrhea is more likely to occur. When diarrhea occurs in a healthy person, unaccompanied by other symptoms, it may be due to the preponderance of bulky fibrous vegetables in tropical diets or to laxative fruits such as figs. In such cases, cutting down of the responsible food may be all that is needed to effect a cure. When there is pain, a feeling of illness and fatigue, discomfort in the abdomen and perhaps bloody discharges, a doctor should be called. These symptoms suggest intestinal infection.

Water lost from the body in perspiration must be replaced. In hot weather thirst usually insures one's drinking enough. Some find it more convenient to drink freely in the cooler parts of the day, when drinks do not bring on so much discomfort from perspiration and prickly heat.

In hot weather the body loses salt as well as water. If the salt needed is not replaced, the chemical processes of the body are disturbed, and there is danger of heat exhaustion, heatstroke, or cramps. One method of supplying this special need of newcomers to the tropics is to add a teaspoonful of table salt to each gallon of drinking water. Others may prefer to take it in tablet form or with their food. It is a mistake to use an excessive amount, producing nausea.

Those accustomed to living in the tropics usually get enough salt in food without supplementing the supply. Acclimated persons lose less salt in perspiration than newcomers. Those engaged in heavy labor, with ensuing excessive perspiration, will do well to use salt tablets with drinking water.

Tea and coffee, taken in moderation, are mild and useful stimulants for most people. They are often the safest available form of refreshment where unboiled water must not be drunk. Excessive indulgence in either can cause insomnia, "nervous heart," and other symptoms of nervousness, however. No permanent injury results, and the cutting down of the amount taken is sufficient for recovery from effects of overstimulation.

The harmful effects of alcohol on the body and the personality cannot be overemphasized. Alcohol is pre-eminently a narcotic, dulling the sensibilities, and not a stimulant as many people think. In regions where loneliness and boredom are common, it is dangerously easy to go to excess in seeking forgetfulness through alcohol or drugs, with a resulting deterioration of health in body and mind which cannot accurately be estimated.

Sleep and Relaxation. Some individuals need more sleep than others. The eight hours usually recommended may not be enough for some adults. Newcomers to the tropics are likely to require more sleep. The siesta is an important part of life in the tropics. Women especially often tire nervously, and they benefit from this break in the strain of the day. The ability to relax mind and body during waking hours is a valuable asset. Many find the reading of light fiction and detective stories a relief from concentration on their work.

In the matter of *exercise,* extremes in either direction are to be avoided. Moderately strenuous setting-up exercises, done habitually in the cool of the morning, provide an excellent way of keeping fit. Outdoor exercise, even if only a walk at sunset, is strongly advised as a daily habit.

The necessity for protecting oneself from the direct rays of the sun is obvious. On the other hand, many people in the tropics go to an extreme, seeking to avoid the sun altogether. A certain amount of *sunshine* or *"skyshine"* is indispensable. In the early morning and late afternoon children should play outdoors. The beneficial effect of the ultraviolet rays from the sun will help in preventing rickets and in building strong, normal bones and teeth.

Bathing indoors is an effective way of cooling off where heat is excessive. Early or late in the day, sea bathing is an excellent form of exercise, improving the circulation and acting as a tonic to the skin. It has been known to cure the persistent crops of boils which are so common at the end of a very hot season. In fresh water one must be careful. Sewage pollution or, in Egypt, North Africa, or Brazil, the presence of snails infected with the fluke disease bilharzia (schistosomiasis) makes streams unsafe for bathing. Bathing water from such places should stand for forty-eight hours to ensure death of parasites. It should be boiled for drinking.

A can of borated talcum powder (10% boric acid) is useful in cases of chafing or prickly heat. Care should be taken to dry the feet thoroughly after bathing. Moisture between the toes encourages the development of athlete's foot. Application of borated talcum powder between the toes is helpful as a preventive. Towels should never be shared with other people, since many skin diseases can be transmitted in that way.

An *annual health examination,* however well one may feel, is to be recommended. At the time of this examination, the doctor can also administer whatever vaccines are due to be repeated.

An annual *vacation* of a month or more, expensive though it may be in terms of time and money, is in the long run a true economy. For some, this holiday will provide the only opportunity for visits to the dentist or the oculist. Mothers and children particularly need a respite from the hot weather.

When circumstances make a journey to a cooler section impracticable, some change of scene can usually be arranged. A visit to friends in a near-by place will provide social contacts and a release from familiar responsibilities. Those who deprive themselves in this respect, although their motive may be unselfish, are likely to defeat their purpose by becoming a burden to their associates through poor health.

It is often when one is physically tired and weak that emotions get out of hand. There is need for understanding how to deal with emotion. Says Dr. Burlingame: [1]"Your emotions are your feelings and, as such, are a driving force which may lead you to great accomplishments. You cannot promise your feelings, but you can promise your behavior. You feel what you feel; know your own feelings, never lie to your own self about them."

Getting Along with Associates

Physical, mental, and what might be called "spiritual" health cannot be separated. Each part of the individual affects the other parts. With emotions accentuated by isolation and the absence of normal avenues of escape from jarring con-

[1] Dr. C. Charles Burlingame, *Rules for Mental Health* (privately printed in Hartford, Conn.).

tacts, one can be made physically ill by misunderstanding, jealousy, and suspicion.

Picture two naturally uncongenial persons closely associated in a lonely station. One, let us say, is consciously troubled by the prospect of further friction between them. His companion is irritable, sarcastic, given to saying things to make one feel inferior and small. The first person is unhappy and miserable. What is he to do?

With a trusted friend at hand, he can talk the situation over, unburden himself of his feelings of hurt and resentment, and hear the viewpoint of an objective person. If there is no such person, he must discuss the matter with himself, ask himself, "Do I really *want* to like this person, have I *tried* to make him like me?" He must examine himself and his habits that others may find annoying or exasperating.

"Am I too talkative, too argumentative or too inquisitive? As an experienced worker, am I bossy, officious, or domineering? As a newcomer, have I begun to think that I know it all? Am I too sensitive, do I read offensive meaning into remarks that are not intended to hurt?" These are questions that one must ask oneself.

He might then go on to a consideration of his associate. To expect perfection is absurd. Minor annoyances must be overlooked in the give and take of living together. When the faults are greater, it may help to try to understand their underlying cause. Abnormal irritability and tension may be due to an over- (or *under-*) active thyroid gland. In such a case, without proper treatment, the person can't help being the way he is.

If you could look into the mind of your associate, too, you might find adequate reason for his behaviour—worries that are all unsuspected, feelings of inferiority and insecurity. A respect for his personality, with sympathy and a genuine desire to like him on your part, may do much toward clearing up the whole difficulty.

There are times when a frank and open discussion can end an unpleasant situation. For this, tact and self-control are necessary. A person who cannot trust himself to keep his temper, will do better to remain silent, to attempt no such discussion. Harsh criticism is likely to destroy any liking your associate may have for you.

Psychology can offer no substitutes for patience and forgiveness. You need live only one minute at a time. And time will pass. Later, when you look back at this period of strain, you will wonder why you found it so upsetting. Realizing this will help you to be patient. And forgive! You simply cannot afford *not* to forgive. Holding a grudge will poison all your thinking and may even make you physically ill.

Make your own life as pleasant for yourself as you can. Avoid unnecessary, continued intimacy with an uncongenial person. Find agreeable companions, and have a room to yourself where you can be alone at times. Take time for rest and recreation every day. Even in those places where human companionship is unavailable, one can relax with hobbies—photography, music, sketching, or making collections of various sorts.

With pets in the tropics one must exercise a certain amount of caution. Rabies, in some parts of India, is quite common. Dogs should be inoculated against it. Ringworm and some other diseases which infect dogs and cats can be transmitted to human beings as well.

SUGGESTED READING

Victor Heiser, M.D., *You're the Doctor,* W. W. Norton & Company, Inc., New York, 1939.

Harold S. Diehl, M.D., *Healthful Living,* McGraw-Hill Book Company, Inc., New York, 1941.

Edward M. Dodd, M.D., *The Health of Our Missions,* Board of Foreign Missions of the Presbyterian Church, New York, 1948.

George H. Preston, M.D., *The Substance of Mental Health,* Rinehart & Company, Inc., New York, 1943.

Smiley Blanton and Norman Vincent Peale, *Faith Is the Answer,* Abingdon-Cokesbury Press, Nashville, Tenn., 1940.

6

WOMEN AND CHILDREN IN THE TROPICS

THE DAY when a country with a hot climate was automatically marked down as "no place for a woman" has passed. There is an increasing demand for women workers in many fields. There is a need for teachers, executives, secretaries, social workers, doctors, nurses, and others with special qualifications.

The happy and well-adjusted wife accompanying her husband to a distant land can glory in her vocation, but it is a grave injustice to take a bride to a life and a country for which she is not fitted. Efficient wifehood under the relatively more exacting conditions in the tropics requires more than usual devotion and ability.

The married woman makes a home for her husband and children; in addition her residence should be a center of social life for the community. In conservative Muslim countries where unchaperoned companionship between men and women is likely to be misunderstood, the home of a married couple provides a place where unmarried associates can enjoy conversation and companionship.

Although she will not as a rule have to do all of her own work, a woman will find that any experience she may have in housekeeping is useful. Even with the uncommon blessing of dependable and well-trained servants, she will have much to do in managing the household. This will require knowledge of local conditions as well as patience and a measure of diplomacy.

Upon arrival the newcomer quickly becomes conscious of one outstanding fact—she cannot speak the language of the country. Even to care for her own family, one must acquire some form of "kitchen dialect." For many this will not be enough. They will employ a teacher or attend a school, and learn to speak and read and write correctly. Such a knowledge is amazingly useful and rewarding.

Children in the Tropics. Normal husbands and wives very naturally want children, but in spite of such a desire they might hesitate to bring children into the world that is the tropics. They may well hesitate, unless they are prepared to give themselves with all their resources to the project of being parents. One must be playmate, parent, teacher, and general mentor. Nurses native to the country, devoted though they may be, are unlikely to teach the child his "Now I lay me down to sleep," or to instruct him in the fundamentals of baseball. The child's thinking must not be allowed to remain at the nurse's level. The child must learn to speak his nation's language without accent. It is to his parents and their friends that he must look for these things.

In remoter sections, the parents' chief problem is that of providing educational facilities for the children. At one time it was a common practice to send the little ones home to boarding school when they reached school age. Relatives or friends could usually be found to care for them during vacations. Now, however, parents are finding means of keeping their children with or *near* them for much longer periods of time. In some cases a mother is the self-appointed teacher, sometimes with the aid of the Calvert or Winnetka systems and children's encyclopedias.[1]

In some cases a mother with teacher's training will enjoy forming a small class of her own children and those of friends. For larger numbers of children, boarding schools have been set up in hill stations and seaside resorts where the climate is good. In some places education is possible even through college years, although many parents prefer transferring their children to schools in their native land before they enter college.

Child Health in the Tropics. Is a child brought up in the

[1] For information write the Calvert School, Baltimore, Maryland, and Winnetka School, Winnetka, Illinois.

tropics handicapped in respect to health? The answer must depend on a number of factors, and the first of these is the parents themselves. Lacking statistics for comparing the number of casualties among children of foreigners in the tropics with those among children of the same nationality brought up in their native land, we can best refer to the report of Dr. Lennox on the results of his study of the children of one foreign group in China. In families where at least one parent had received education in medicine or nursing, the child death rate was only about two-thirds of that in families where there was no such training. It is, then, only reasonable to infer that the physical welfare of children in hot climates is proportionate to their parent's skill in taking care of them.

There is, of course, the factor of varying climates and disease risks. Some places are associated with greater risks than are others. Angola, in western Africa, was long considered as almost certainly fatal for foreign children remaining there beyond the age of infancy. Within recent years, however, as a result of efficient methods of disease prevention and increased knowledge regarding nutrition, Angola has been found safe for children.

The Child's Nurse. To help in the care of small children, a nurse from among the people of the country is usually available. Some of these have had experience in other families, and are loyal and trustworthy in every respect. In other places, the mother must choose a clean, healthy woman or girl and train her.

A nurse can be invaluable in a hot climate where the mother needs some degree of freedom for health's sake. After the baby is bathed and fed, the nurse can at least wheel him out in his carriage for a longer time than the mother can spare from her other duties. She can watch over the older children in their play, do all the routine work of keeping the nursery clean, and act as baby sitter when the mother and father go out to dinner in the evening.

It is important that anyone caring for children should be healthy. An examination, including if possible X-ray of the chest for tuberculosis, blood tests for syphilis, and a stool examination for dysentery germs, should be made. The doctor should certify that the nurse is free from venereal diseases of all kinds, that she does not have trachoma or other contagious diseases of the eyes or skin.

To insure the cleanliness of servants having close contact with the family, it is a good plan to provide new clothing to be worn only at work. Inspection of the hair for vermin, with suitable treatment when needed, is a very practical concern. It will be a great advantage if a bathroom can be set apart where the nurse can take a bath on coming to work.

The nurse must always be carefully supervised. Take nothing for granted. Such servants often come from a society where it is usual to give opium to babies to keep them from crying. They have little understanding of hygiene as we know it, regarding flies as a minor irritation rather than as possible transmitters of eye disease or intestinal infections. The well-trained nurse may be exemplary in all these respects but, even so, she must not be left entirely to her own devices.

The child's nurse is usually sincerely devoted to the children under her care, and they often love her fondly in return. Unfortunately, her devotion may have some unfortunate influence on little folk. She may, through mistaken adoration, assume the attitude of slave and encourage the little master or mistress to give orders which should be permitted only to parents. A child becoming imperious and striking his nurse when she fails to please is not to be tolerated. An attitude of respectful consideration on the part of the children toward all the servants should be instilled in them very early.

Boys and girls need work, just as adults do. Daily chores are essential, and may not be easy to invent in a household where servants do the work. For play, swings and seesaws, sand piles and play houses are easy to build. Simple improvised toys are wonderful for children.

Love is the sunshine in which little lives unfold. Impersonal care, however efficient, cannot take its place. The security of family life, individual attention, and discipline—which is a manifestation of love and firm but never harsh—are necessary if the child is to thrive.

7

A HOME IN THE TROPICS

▀▄

As a rule the traveler finds his future residence already prepared by those who have preceded him. An overcritical attitude will avail him nothing. Such innovations as he might like to make may be entirely out of the question or impracticable. Later he may have an opportunity to build his own dream house. From a study of considerations which are important in building a house, he may find suggestions for improving the place in which he lives.

In the selection of a home site, there are several factors to consider. The most obvious of these is perhaps that of comfort. The prospective builder will consider prevailing winds, to have the full benefit of cooling breezes. The health aspects of the site must be given careful consideration, too. Natural drainage is to be noted. Standing water or swampy ground provides breeding places for mosquitoes. Therefore a high spot on a slope is desirable. Proximity of villages with high malaria rates must be investigated. Infected mosquitoes can fly a mile.

As a foundation sand makes a better base than clay, which tends to undergo changes, with cracking walls as a result. The location of ground water must be ascertained. For this a depth of six to eight feet in all seasons is best. The availability of good, abundant drinking water is a primary need. Surface water—in streams, ponds, and the like—may almost always be assumed to be polluted. Ground water—that which is brought to the surface in springs and wells—may be heavily infected, however clear and sparkling it may appear. When testing of the water by means of specimens sent to a public health laboratory is impossible, it is safer to take it for granted that the water requires boiling before use.

Where wells, whether shallow or artesian, are to be drilled, an impervious cover of concrete, as well as a casing of the same material should be arranged. The casing should rise at least eighteen inches above the ground and go as far as possible down into the well, preferably one foot below the lowest ground-water level.

Rain water to be used for drinking purposes should be caught on a clean, waterproof surface. In houses with a central court the roof is used for this purpose, with a funnel of sail cloth attached to catch the overflow. All cisterns or tanks for water should be watertight and covered, with a direct overflow outside. Screen all openings to prevent mosquitoes' breeding.

Underbrush should be cleared away from about the house to a distance of at least ten feet since it provides a place of concealment for snakes and mosquitoes. Vines growing on the house give shelter to vermin.

Screening the house, and especially the bedrooms, is very important and doors and windows should be constructed with this in view. All openings should be arranged so as to provide the maximum circulation of air. The beauties and advantages of local styles of architecture should not be lightly ignored.

Building materials will vary according to local resources. Thick adobe walls, popular in many places, exclude the heat effectively. Cement, however, is coming into more general use because it is proof against rats and termites. Also, its light color absorbs little heat. When cement is used, walls should extend about two feet below the surface of the ground. All openings, of course, should be screened. Rats are particularly dangerous in regions where epidemics of plague occur.

Termites are a common and constant menace in tropical parts. Where cement is not used for construction, other measures can be taken for protection of building materials used. A horizontal sheet of galvanized iron with edges turned down can be incorporated into foundations or posts on which the building rests. The steps to a house need not actually touch the building, and termites will not be able to cross the gap. The kind of wood most resistant to termites should be selected.

A chemical wash of crude creosote, plymol, or solignum, used as a coating on wooden parts is another means of protection. Piles of timber should not be left in the vicinity of houses.

A mixture which is effective against white ants is given by Stitt. Two pounds of dry commercial arsenic is mixed with two pounds of dry commercial caustic soda. Add two gallons of water slowly, since the mixing produces much heat and may cause the mixture to boil over. The resulting paste is boiled for a few minutes with continued stirring and then cooled and strained through clean hessian (hemp) or similar material. It can then be bottled, labeled *POISON*, and stored for use.

This solution may be applied to surfaces of floors, walls, or furniture, but it is best to test it before extensive use. Wood that has already been attacked by the ants can be treated by applying the solution to the ant tunnels and surrounding wood or by boring auger holes diagonally downward and filling the holes with the liquid.

In some tropical communities air conditioning is available. The difference between indoor and outdoor temperature should not be allowed to exceed 10 to 15 degrees. Insulation against heat can be provided by including aluminum foil in the walls. The punkah, a long fan of straw matting slung from the ceiling, has long been used in India. A swaying motion is given to the fan by means of a rope pulled by a servant on the veranda. Electric fans have been introduced in many places.

The khus-khus tattie, inserted in windows and doors, consists of a layer of fiber or roots between two sheets of metal screening. The fiber is kept wet so that air coming into the room is cooled by evaporation of the water.

For warmth in the cool season fireplaces may help.

Flat roofs of clay, surrounded by a parapet are common in some countries and are often used for sleeping purposes in hot weather. These are likely to leak unless they are repaired before the rainy season. Where rain is excessive a sloping roof is needed. Thatched roofs harbor vermin.

Sanitary toilet facilities must be provided not only for members of the family, but for those employed in the house. While modern toilet facilities are becoming increasingly common in many places the system of placing individual commodes in bathrooms is still used. With efficient scavenger service, the pails are emptied and washed several times during each day. Sanitary privies and bore-hole latrines are used in some places. The latter is a device suitable for use over a limited period of time and in locations where the ground water is not too near the surface. Its construction is inexpensive and when one hole has been filled another can be drilled. The apparatus can be carried in a car for touring. An augur fourteen to sixteen inches in diameter is used to bore a hole eight to twenty feet deep. A perforated slab made to fit over the hole constitutes the floor of the toilet. All privies and latrines should be located at least fifty feet away from the residence or any well.

Better than either the commode system or the use of privies is the practice of having toilets empty into a septic tank. In it the contents are changed and rendered harmless and colorless by bacteria, favored by darkness, stillness, and the absence of air. A few shovelfuls of horse manure added now and then will prevent odor and clogging. When the process of change is complete the resulting fluid is suitable for use in irrigation.

Exposed garbage not only favors the breeding of flies but also attracts rats. Bottles and tin cans, unless crushed and flattened, collect rain water in which mosquitoes breed. Refuse may be either burned or buried. Composting all refuse by burying it twelve to eighteen inches beneath the surface of the ground will provide, in years to come, a very fertile spot for gardening.

J. Balfour Kirk, *A Manual of Sanitation*, Bailliere, Tindall and Cox, London.
For sale by Superintendent of Documents, Washington, D.C.:
The Sanitary Privy, Supp. 108, Public Health Report, 5¢.
Sewage Disposal for Suburban and Country Homes, Supp. 58, Public Health Report, 10¢.
Sewage and Garbage Disposal on the Farm, Farmers' Bulletin 1950, 10¢.
Obtainable from Virginia State Dept. of Health, Richmond:
Septic Tanks for Suburban and Country Homes: Built-in-Place Concrete Septic Tanks (1941).
The Sanitary Pit Privy (1941).

8

HOUSEHOLD PRECAUTIONS

THE IMPORTANCE of safe drinking water cannot be overemphasized. Except where the municipal supply is adequately chlorinated, all water to be used for drinking, brushing the teeth, or for finger bowls should be boiled for five minutes. A large pot or kettle with a cover makes a good container. The ladle used for removing the contents should be sterilized and allowed to stand in the pot. One cannot always depend on servants to attend to this.

Unclean water requires filtering *before* boiling, not after. And filtering alone does not make water safe for drinking. The Berkfield filter has a capacity usually sufficient for household use. It should be cleaned twice a week, and since the cylinders are rather fragile a soft brush is used to remove the film which collects on them. When the cylinders are clean, they are placed in cold water which is brought slowly to a boil and, after 15 minutes' boiling, allowed to stand for gradual cooling.

When filtration is impracticable, the sediment in water can be settled by the addition of a pinch of alum. After the alum has acted for 15 or 20 minutes, the clear water may be poured off for boiling, leaving the sediment in the bottom of the container. For large quantities of muddy water ⅓ grain of alum is needed for each gallon. If the water is soft this amount of alum will render it acid. In such a case ⅓ grain of washing soda should be added to the water for each grain of alum used.

Water should be not only safe and clear but cool. Unless ice is known to be made of safe water it should not be added to drinks. Bottles of boiled water can be placed around a block of ice, however. A device common in the tropics is that of keeping drinking water in a porous earthen jar, placed in the breeze to promote evaporation. After a jar is washed and scalded, when new, a handful of salt thrown into it and washed out after a few hours will increase its cooling power. The mouth of the jar should, of course, be covered to protect it from dust.

Water may be made safe for drinking by the addition of certain chemicals. *Chlorinated lime* is commonly used for this purpose. One pound of good grade chlorinated lime (dry) is mixed with a half gallon of water to make a stock solution. One teaspoonful of this solution is added to each gallon of drinking water. After fifteen minutes, provided there is a slight taste or odor of chlorine, the water may be used.

For disinfecting a well of ordinary size, dissolve 2 glassfuls of dry chloride of lime in a pail of water, strain through muslin, and pour into the well.

Halazone tablets, containing chlorine, are useful while one is traveling. Since these tablets deteriorate rapidly on exposure, they should be bottled in quantities of not more than 100. One tablet is usually sufficient for a quart or liter of water. Hard tablets should be crushed in a piece of paper before use, and water should stand for half an hour after being stirred or shaken in a bottle. An odor of chlorine is an indication that enough of the chemical has been added.

Tablets of *sodium bisulphate* are marketed for use of travelers. For one pint of water, 15 grains is required. Vessels of aluminum are suitable for this solution, but not those of copper or iron. It does not keep well and should be freshly made.

One drop of 7.5 per cent *tincture of iodine* will sterilize a quart of water. Water should stand for 15 minutes before use.

Potassium permanganate is useful against cholera germs but is *not* a reliable antiseptic for killing dysentery germs. On the whole, chlorine is a more reliable agent, even for cholera germs.

Boiling or Pasteurization of Milk. Fresh milk, from whatever animal, can seldom be guaranteed to be safe without boiling or pasteurization. Even with careful handling of the animal by a healthy individual, with examination of livestock to insure against undulant (Malta) fever and tuberculosis, there is still a chance that milk may be contaminated by the vessel in which it is collected or the hands of the milker. The slight advantages of raw milk are far outweighed by its disadvantages.

Boiling milk 1 to 3 minutes in an open saucepan, with stirring, is the simplest method of killing disease germs. When using a double boiler one should extend the time to 10 or 20 minutes after water in the bottom pan has begun to boil. Pasteurization consists in heating milk or cream to a temperature of 145° F. and keeping it at that point for 30 minutes. In *flash pasteurization,* the milk is brought to a boil, taken immediately from the fire, and the pan surrounded by ice or very cold water.

Butter and cheese made of unsafe milk can transmit disease. When making these products in the home, one can pasteurize the milk or cream used. Doubtfully safe butter and cheese can be pasteurized in the top of a double boiler. They will melt but solidify again on cooling. In many places reliable brands of canned butter are available. Canned, sterilized, and dried milk are very useful in the tropics. Relatively small cans are preferable since the contents of larger sizes may spoil before they are used.

Food Safety. A large proportion of the diseases common in the tropics are due to contamination of food or drink with disease germs which can be destroyed by heat. In most cases the usual cooking time is sufficient for foods, but pork must be cooked 30 minutes for every pound of weight, to guard against trichinosis. This procedure will also protect one from pork tape worm. Where beef tape worm occurs, beef must also be thoroughly cooked. The same applies to fish, crayfish, and crabs which in some localities are frequently infected with certain fluke diseases.

Perishable foods such as meat and sea food must be purchased very fresh and preferably in amounts to be eaten during one meal. They should be cooked and eaten without delay.

Foods of the custard type—cream puffs and ice cream—often give rise to epidemics of food poisoning, since germs from hands or throats of food handlers multiply rapidly in them. Leftovers must not be allowed to accumulate and food should not be placed in direct contact with ice. It must be understood that freezing does *not* kill germs; it merely delays their action.

Canned foods are valuable food resources in the tropics. When cans bulge, or emit a hollow sound on being tapped, there is a possibility of spoilage. More than two solder marks on the can indicate that it has been opened and resealed. Whenever the contents of tins seem abnormal in color, consistency, odor, or taste, it is safer to discard them. Although germs in the contents would be destroyed by boiling, poisonous substances are not so removed.

The preparation of raw fruits and vegetables requires the housekeeper's personal attention, especially where dysentery is a common complaint. Only when it is certain that human excreta have not been used as fertilizer can one depend on the usual washing and scrubbing to make these foods safe. Washing fruits and salad vegetables with potassium permanganate is *not* sufficient, since this does not destroy germs of dysentery. An effective method, worked out by doctors in China is to dip each piece in briskly boiling water, for a period of 10 seconds. For fruits with rough or irregular surfaces, 20 seconds is recommended. Most fruits will not be much changed by this process. Lettuce will be wilted but usable after chilling.

Melons, as we have mentioned, may have been made to absorb unsafe water to increase their weight. Water has at times been injected into persimmons by means of a hypodermic syringe for the same purpose. Immersing them in boiling water, even for 20 seconds, would not make such fruits safe, of course.

Cleanliness in the kitchen is essential. Unhealthy or unclean food handlers are a definite menace. A cook harboring dysentery germs can infect the whole household through his fingers. When possible, the stools of all food handlers should be examined twice a year. Those in whom infection is discovered should be suspended from all work associated with food until pronounced cured by a doctor. Train all servants to wash their hands carefully before touching food. Provide soap and water for that purpose. When dishes have been washed, the most sanitary practice is to pour boiling water over them and allow them to dry by evaporation. In any case, dirty dish towels are not to be tolerated.

Protection from Insects. Flies are so common in hot countries that the natives adopt a philosophic attitude toward them. Some Arabs, for example, have a tradition that while flies carry harm on one wing, they carry benefit on the other.

Modern science is not so sanguine about them. The housefly, we find, breeds by preference in human excreta, and it can fly as far as eleven miles in four days. Before eating food, it deposits any germs it may have eaten. This undoubtedly explains many cases of dysentery, typhoid fever, and other intestinal diseases.

The potential danger of houseflies needs to be understood; at the same time, too much thinking about them may lead to harmful worry which accomplishes nothing helpful. A sensible and practical attitude, combined with habitual carefulness, is infinitely better. The use of screening, the spraying every two or three months with DDT of walls and other places where flies light, daily use of the spray gun and the fly swatter, and careful training of servants do much to reduce the hazards. Cloth covers, like doilies of cotton net weighted with a bead fringe, are often used for covering the milk pitcher, honey jar, and other such dishes.

Mosquitoes carry some of the most dreaded of tropical diseases, including malaria and yellow fever. When metal screening for the home is unavailable, cotton netting can be tacked over the windows and draped to curtain the doors. Standing water about the house should be eliminated. Water in the saucers of flower pots, in empty coconut shells, tin cans, hollow trees, hoof prints, and the cupped leaves of trees and plants may provide a breeding place for some varieties. Roof gutters must be kept clear during the rainy season to prevent water from collecting on the roof.

Every member of the family should have his own bed net.

Cotton netting with a mesh of sixteen or eighteen threads to the inch should be used for these. In one common type the netting forms a cubicle about the bed. The rectangular top, exactly the size of the mattress, has tapes sewn to its corners for attachment to posts at the corners of the bedstead. The four walls of netting, extending about four feet above the mattress, may have a foot of muslin or canvas at the bottom to tuck under the mattress. Some people prefer to have canvas extend a foot above the mattress to prevent mosquitoes from biting the sleeper if he lies against the netting.

Constant watchfulness is needed for discovery and repair of holes in bed nets, as is a morning and evening inspection and spraying with insecticide in case mosquitoes have been imprisoned. Nets are folded over the top of the posts in the morning, and tucked in all around the mattress at about sundown. In going to bed, one pulls out the margin just enough to get inside, then quickly tucks it in again. Provision of a flap, like a door, is *not* advisable.

Malarial mosquitoes, which bite only at night, can often be swatted while resting on walls in the daytime. DDT sprayed on walls acts slowly but has a lasting effect. It is said that electric lights or storm lanterns placed under dinner tables during meals prevent mosquitoes from coming to bite the ankles of diners. The expedient of burning punk or incense is well known, too.

DDT (dichlorodiphenyl-trichloroethane!) is a recent and effective insecticide. Insoluble in water, it can be used as a solution in oil, as an emulsion diluted with water, or in combination with a dusting powder. Its outstanding characteristic is its *prolonged* poisonous effect. It does not act so quickly as Flit.

DDT is practically useless unless properly applied. The average user should buy prepared products. Such preparations indicate on the label the percentage of DDT and have explicit directions for use. Emulsions are best for general use, since they can be stored in concentrated form and diluted with water as needed. They dry more quickly than kerosene solutions, create less fire hazard, have little odor, and leave no objectionable stain when lightly applied. They should not, however be used on varnished surfaces.

Oil solutions and emulsions may be painted on a surface or used as a spray. Painting of door and window screens is economical and effective. For penetrating cracks, DDT solution or emulsion can be squirted with an oil can.

Used as a spray indoors, a 5 per cent solution or emulsion of DDT is toxic to anopheles mosquitoes for several months, as well as houseflies. Outside, even a ½ per cent DDT emulsion or solution applied to fly breeding places will kill the flies as they emerge for about three weeks. In the home, care must be taken that flies killed by the insecticide do not fall into milk or food.

Two ounces of talcum powder containing 10 per cent DDT will control body lice on the individual. Garments should be dusted most carefully about the seams. After such treatment clothing may be washed once and still remain lice free. For bedbugs a 5 per cent emulsion or solution, used as a spray on infested beds and walls and floors about beds will give complete protection for six months at least. Bugs may remain alive for forty-eight hours after the spraying, and for quick results a spray containing pyrethrum may be used at the same time.

A 5 per cent or 10 per cent emulsion of DDT applied to walls, ceiling, and floors, with close attention given to cracks and dark corners, is partially effective against cockroaches. A week after the spraying, dusting powder containing 10 per cent DDT should be applied to cracks and crevices. Spraying and dusting will need to be repeated at regular intervals, since the insecticide has little or no toxic effects on the eggs of insects.

To control fleas, a 5 per cent emulsion of DDT should be applied to floors and rugs of infested rooms and to basements. Animals' sleeping baskets should also be sprayed, but the animals should not. A 5 per cent or 10 per cent DDT dusting powder may be used for dogs, a third of an ounce being enough for a medium-sized dog. Cats lick their fur and for this reason DDT should not be used on them.

Spiders, crickets, carpet beetles, ants, centipedes, moths, silverfish, and other household pests are killed by DDT. Expert opinion should be obtained, however, before using it to eliminate agricultural pests, lest plant tissue be harmed and beneficial insects and parasites be destroyed.

DDT can be handled without danger provided there is no constant or excessive exposure of the skin to *oil solutions*. The emulsions or kerosene solutions should never be allowed to remain on the skin or saturate clothing. After using such preparations, wash the hands with soap and water, and when work is completed, a soapy bath should be taken. For occasional spraying work, wear old clothes and remove them when the work is done. For regular residual spraying, a chemical cartridge respirator, goggles, rubber gloves, and heavy clothes and hat should be worn. If skin or eyes become inflamed from DDT sprays, treat affected parts with a warm solution of boric acid until a doctor can be consulted or relief is obtained. When DDT is swallowed, give mustard water (1 tablespoonful of powdered mustard to a glass of warm water) to induce vomiting. A physician should be called.

Probably the best insect repellent for keeping off mosquitoes, gnats, flies, etc., is that known as 6–2–2 mixture. It is effective against a wide variety of insects. A half teaspoonful is poured in the palm of the hand, one then rubs the hands together and applies a thin layer to the face, neck, ears, hands, and wrists. It may also be sprayed or rubbed on clothing.[1]

During protracted rainy seasons, leather goods often become moldy and need to be wiped dry every day. Contents of clothes closets should be hung out in the sunshine at every opportunity during such a season. An electric bulb burning in a closet helps to prevent mold. One kind of fungus growth causes stains resembling iron rust on bed and table linen and clothing. Sprinkling formaldehyde solution on the fabrics or placing small bags of formaldehyde on shelves where such articles are stored will destroy these air-borne fungi.

[1] For further information see Miscellaneous Publication No. 606, U.S. Department of Agriculture, entitled *DDT and Other Insecticides and Repellents.*

9

SERVANTS IN THE TROPICS

SOME PERSONS come to the tropics fully intending to manage their homes without the help of servants. It is wise to familiarize oneself with local conditions before too fully resolving upon such a course of action.

In parts of India and along the Persian Gulf the usual kitchen is a crude structure separate from the house. Water is carried from the well. The kitchen stove, built of clay, is designed to burn wood or charcoal. The oven, placed on the stove when in use, resembles a huge pillbox with a fire burning on the cover.

Even providing that one is willing to defy custom to the extent of making the daily marketing trip to the food bazaar in company with the neighbors' cooks, the exertion in the heat of the day is exhausting. One is at a disadvantage in the customary bargaining for food. A hired cook can get better values at a much lower price. Even when he takes a small commission for himself, the employer is still saving money on the transaction, as a rule.

The caste system in India permits the individual servant to do only his own particular kind of work. The resultant multiplicity of helpers is reflected in neighboring countries, among them Arabia, where the caste system does not prevail. One manservant will cook, another washes clothes, another carries water, while still another does the scavenging work necessitated by the commode system in bathrooms.

The dhobi who brings back the laundry looking so clean and

43

neat can usually be shared with other families. The same is true of the man who does the bathroom work, as well as the water carrier. But in most homes, the cook's service is supplemented by another servant who serves the food and keeps the house in order. Where there are children, employment of a nurse is taken for granted.

The expense involved in the employment of so many servants is not nearly so terrifying as it might be thought. Wages in tropical countries are very low. It may be less expensive to live in this way in a rural part of the country than to rent an apartment with modern conveniences in a large city, where fewer servants are the rule.

One cannot live in the tropics for any length of time without realizing how much established custom governs the life of everyone there. To some extent this is true elsewhere, but in the tropics it seems that what is, has always been, and must forever be. A man will sooner give up his job than do a thing that is not customarily done by the people of his caste. In matters related to caste and religion, one can only bow to necessity.

This state of affairs is not always a disadvantage to the employer. Fair and considerate employers have preceded him, and he need only fit into the established pattern. He can make innovations, of course, which are pleasing to his helpers, such as allowing them longer leaves of absence during religious holidays. But in doing so he must realize that he will find it difficult to change what becomes so easily an established precedent. It is well to confer with friends and neighbors before initiating a change.

Life is certainly made easier and pleasanter when one has servants. The poor people about one are given needed employment and one is given an opportunity to concentrate more fully on his own work. But with these advantages come certain responsibilities. The importance of selecting healthy food handlers and nurses has been stressed elsewhere. There are other factors, too, that must be considered.

The management and training of helpers with a background so foreign to the employer's own experience require special qualifications on his part. Dr. J. G. Vaughan, contributes the following advice on the subject:

For the first year it is well to live in a home entirely or at least partly managed by one who knows the people and their language. The entire housekeeping ménage will probably be quite different from anything experienced in the past; the foods and their seasons, the market prices, the method of preparation, the kitchen and housekeeping equipment and technique, the temper and frailties of servants are all matters well worth learning from one who has had much experience. Be patient and take time to learn these important lessons. Servants are great blessings and can bring comfort and order to the home and relieve the mistress of the home of all the drudgery. But first know well yourself the job you want your servants to do and then learn the frailties and foibles as well as the strength and capacity of your servants. The wise woman is she who is mistress of her own kitchen, and by her intelligent understanding of this basic center of the family health commands the respect and obedient cooperation of her servants.

But these helpers, so necessary in the tropics, are sometimes the most vexing problem that the newcomer has to face. Usually with the help of older workers in your vicinity you will find one or two servants who have some skill and experience in the work of the foreigner's home. May it be your good fortune to find one of those "jewels" who by their skill and loyalty carry faithfully their important responsibilities. But it is quite possible you will not be so fortunate. Unless trained for many years in foreign households the native servant has an all too inadequate understanding of hygiene and sanitation, and perhaps of simple cleanliness as we know it. In countries where the various dysenteric diseases and other microbic infections are ever present, the wise and skillful mistress will be eternally vigilant in her supervision. Even in such a simple process as boiling milk and drinking water you must be sure from constant observance of his technique that your cook can be trusted. Your skill or lack of it, in securing efficient service in respect to these two items, namely, sterilization of water and milk, may mean the difference between sickness and health for the members of your household. They [your servants] come from a background of poverty, as a rule, and their wages are very paltry judged by Western standards. Careless supervision encourages dishonesty and theft. Usually they sense a moral code of their own that makes for great faithfulness and trustworthiness when specifically assigned responsibility for safeguarding the property of their mistress. But it must be mutually understood by both mistress and servant that an inventory has been made and is being constantly checked. Skill in doing this without loss of "face" for the servant and yet letting him know that you are watching the faithfulness with which he discharges his stewardship will encourage his honesty and loyalty. Many a servant of honest intentions is made dishonest by a careless and shiftless mistress.

It is indeed true that some good household helpers are spoiled by their employers' shortcomings. A good beginning is very important to a successful relationship. Servants are watching to see what sort of a person this new master or mistress will be. Be sure to get a reputation from the beginning for being particular. An impression of laxness cannot later be changed without a great deal of unpleasantness. Never pass over even a small neglect of duty. Quietly, without any display of temper insist on obedience in every detail. Whether supplies are to be kept under lock and key will depend upon circumstances. In some places this is a necessary precaution. Be considerate and fair in your dealings with servants. Do not be afraid to show an interest in their affairs and the welfare of their families. But never be undignified or too talkative about trivial affairs. Otherwise what is meant for a democratic spirit is likely to be misunderstood as weakness.

The employment of servants is far from being an unmixed luxury. To take unpromising material and produce an efficient and reliable helper may be an exacting task. But the employer who can teach those who serve him to be valuable assistants, well trained and unspoiled, makes an important contribution to his own household, to future employers, and also to the servant himself.

10

FOOD AND HEALTH

▀▀

PART I

Revised by Mary Katharine Russell, M.S.

"WHAT DID YOU have to eat over there?" Of all the questions asked of people returning from the tropics this is probably the most frequent. Those who have stayed at home expect to find great changes in their friends who have lived in far-off parts of the world. They may be surprised to find them normal individuals who apparently have not suffered from undernourishment.

When trying to answer a question of this sort a person recalls many things. Sometimes his mouth waters at the thought of juicy mangoes, succulent fresh figs, and dates newly ripened on the date palm, luscious fruit which slip out of the skin like a concord grape. Maybe he thinks with longing of the water chestnuts, bean sprouts, and Chinese cabbage so well cooked in Chinese food, of the flavor of chillies in Mexican dishes or of spicy curries enjoyed in India. To prove how enjoyable tropical foods can be he may invite his friends to some local restaurant where his favorite exotic dishes are served.

The majority of travelers will find at their journey's end the possibility of getting many of the foods to which they are accustomed. However, he who has the true spirit of adventure will find, in addition, many new and exciting dietary

47

experiences awaiting him in the far corners of the world, and if he is alert he will want to know how these foods can contribute to the nutritive value, as well as to the interest, of his own table. In many places, the newcomer may have a garden. Here he may introduce foods, familiar to him but new to the locality, which may enrich the diet of the local people. In this way, tomatoes were introduced by an agriculturist and are grown now by many people in a section of North China. The one who is truly wise and truly friendly will find that the learning process is a two-way street, and that in foods and nutrition, as in other fields, he has much to learn and at the same time he can share what he knows.

Persons who plan to live in a foreign land have a special need for knowing just what is important concerning foods. Those who will bear the responsibility for their own health and that of others should whenever possible avail themselves of a course in nutrition or at least provide themselves with literature on the subject.[1]

THE BODY'S NEEDS

THE BODY uses food (1) to supply energy; (2) to build and repair body tissues; and (3) to regulate body processes. The first need is supplied by carbohydrates, fats, and proteins. Proteins, minerals, and water build and repair tissues. The body processes are regulated by water, proteins, minerals, vitamins, and bulk, or roughage. Each of these, except roughage, is a nutrient group. But each group contains many different nutrients. Proteins are made up of twenty-two amino acids, of which at least eight or ten must be present in our foods. We have specific use for at least thirteen minerals—perhaps more. Scientists have studied many of the substances called vitamins, which occur in such minute amounts and yet are so important. Fifteen vitamins may be necessary for the well-being of the human body. Four of these are soluble in fat and eleven in water. We must have food which will furnish glucose to the

[1] See suggested readings at the end of the chapter.

body, and some highly unsaturated fatty acid seems to be nutritionally essential. Our daily diet need not be checked for the presence of all these nutrients, however. For example, some of the vitamins are probably produced in sufficient quantity in the healthy intestinal tract and need not be present in the food under normal conditions. Others are "trailer" nutrients, which come along with another essential, for example, sulfur, which is a constituent of protein.

To simplify the task of planning the day's meals the following pattern has been suggested.

A GUIDE FOR AN ADEQUATE DAILY DIET FOR THE FAMILY [2]

MILK

Recommended amounts:
1 quart for each child and each prospective mother
1½ quarts for each nursing mother
3 or 4 cups for each adult
Minimum amounts:
3 or 4 cups for each child
1 quart for each prospective mother
1½ quarts for each nursing mother
2 or 3 cups for each adult

FRUITS
1 serving of fresh citrus fruit such as orange or grapefruit or a serving of tomatoes, raw or canned
1 serving of other fruit, fresh or dried, cooked or raw

VEGETABLES
1 or more servings of potato
2 or more servings of other vegetables, at least one of which should be of the green or yellow varieties

[2] Taken from *Recommended Dietary Allowance*, National Research Council, Reprint and Circular Series, Number 115, January, 1943. Copies of this pamphlet or later editions may be obtained without charge on request from the Food and Nutrition Board, National Research Council, 2101 Constitution Avenue, Washington 25, D.C.

EGGS
> *Recommended amount:* 1 egg for each child and each adult
> (occasionally 2 eggs for adults)
> *Minimum amount:* 3 or 4 eggs a week for each person

LEAN MEAT, FISH OR OTHER SEA-FOOD
AND POULTRY
> *Recommended amount:* 1 or sometimes 2 servings daily
> *Minimum amounts:*
> 1 serving on at least 5 days a week
> On days when meat is not served dried beans, dried peas, peanut
> butter, nuts, cheese, or eggs may be substituted

CEREALS AND BREADS (*whole grain or "enriched" with thiamin*)
> *Cereal:* 1 serving daily
> *Bread:* 1 serving at each meal (more bread may need to be eaten
> if the requirement for energy is unusual or if for some reason
> other foods are limited)

FATS AND SUGARS
> *Butter:* 1 tablespoonful (or the same amount of oleomargarine,
> to which vitamin A has been added)
> *Sugars and fats other than butter:* as needed for energy

Most readers can make available for themselves and their families a large proportion of the foods here suggested for an adequate diet. Where certain foods are not available, substitutions may be made, but care must be taken that the foods which are substituted contain all the nutrients that would have been furnished by the items omitted. For example, if no animal milk can be obtained, soybean or peanut milk might be substituted. It would be comparatively simple to supply in soybeans and peanuts the needed quantity of protein (though, as we shall see, the quality may be in question). But have precautions been taken to provide the calcium which would have been found in the animal milk? Here a glance at the table of nutritive values (Appendix A, III) will supply the answer.

This diet guide presents an "American style" pattern. Other

satisfactory patterns can be substituted, using local foodstuffs. This project should be a matter of study.

WHAT ARE THE classes of nutrients to be considered in planning a diet? *Water* is the first essential, and its lack is the most critical. The body may lose all its reserves of fat and half its protein without serious danger, but the loss of 10 per cent of the water of the body is serious, and the loss of 20 per cent may be fatal.

Bulk, or *roughage,* while not technically a nutrient because it is not absorbed by the body, is important as it assists in the digestion of food and in maintaining the health of the intestinal tract.

Carbohydrates (*Starches and Sugars*)

Bread, cereals, starchy vegetables like potatoes, sweet vegetables, fruits, sugar, and syrups come in this classification. Carbohydrates are the cheapest source of food energy and are usually eaten in large amounts in tropical countries; but varieties associated with important minerals and vitamins are sometimes not available.

Fats

These, with carbohydrates and proteins, constitute the *energy-producing food materials.* Fats produce more than twice as much food energy as do corresponding weights of carbohydrate or protein foods. A certain amount of fat is needed everywhere not only to contribute calories for energy, especially for the needs of very active persons, but also to make food palatable. For energy and palatability, animal fats (including the fat of meat and lard) and vegetable fats (like coconut, olive, peanut, and cottonseed oil) are equally useful. Cream, butter, some fish oils, and the oil of the red palm also contribute vitamin A as does enriched oleomargarine.

Oils, such as olive or peanut oil, available locally and relatively inexpensive, may be as valuable nutritionally as more expensive solid fats. Fatty foods or foods cooked in fats are often spoken of as "difficult to digest," but what is really meant, in the case of healthy adults, is that they are slower in digestion than some other foods. Therein lies one of their special contributions: because they are slower of digestion they help to keep us from being hungry before time for the next meal.

Concerning the *amount* of fat needed, the Food and Nutrition Board of the National Research Council (after this referred to as the Food and Nutrition Board) recommends that (1) fat be included in the diet to the extent of at least 20 to 25 per cent of the total calories and (2) that the fat intake include essential unsaturated fatty acids (found in natural fats) to the extent of at least 1 per cent of the total calories. For very active persons consuming 4500 calories and for children and adolescents it is considered desirable that 30 to 35 per cent of total calories be derived from fat. Since foodstuffs such as meat, milk, cheese, nuts, and the like contribute fat to the diet, it is necessary to use separated or "visible" fats such as butter, oleomargarine, lard, or shortenings to supply only one-third to one-half the amounts indicated.

Proteins

Besides producing energy, proteins are of great importance as *building foods*. In many cases the need for supplying protein of good quality is the most difficult problem facing people with low income. Not all proteins are equally valuable. Of the twenty-two amino acids which make up the proteins of the body, at least eight must be present in the food of the ordinary adult. Some others can be built up in the body, but not these, and so we call these the "essential" amino acids. There is evidence that still others cannot be built rapidly enough to supply the body's needs in periods of rapid growth (such as infancy and childhood, pregnancy, and lactation), so then they, too, become "essential." A protein which supplies all the "essential" amino acids in suitable proportions is a "high-quality," or "complete," protein; if it lacks even one, or possesses it in too small a quantity, it is of lesser value to the body.

Pre-eminent among the most useful proteins are those of *animal* origin: meat, fowl, fish and other sea foods, eggs, milk, and cheese. Unfortunately animal proteins are the most expensive of foods and often out of reach for the poor. Also, vegetarians, as in the case of the Hindu people, are prohibited from consuming any animal foods excepting milk and cheese and, in some instances, eggs.[3]

Tiny, dried fish furnish the only animal protein in some communities while in other places people prevent ill effects from deficiency of animal protein by eating locusts, grasshoppers, caterpillars, grubs found in the pith of palm trees, and the eggs of termites.

Of the *vegetable* foods, soybeans and peanuts contain proteins more closely approximating in value those from animal sources. Soybeans are much used in China. Peanuts roasted and eaten plain are suitable for adults. For children they are a valuable food when made into peanut butter. To make this, roasted peanuts (also called "monkey nuts" or "ground nuts") are put six to eight times through a meat grinder, using a fine blade. Nothing is added except salt to taste, or a little peanut or other oil if a softer product is desired.

Other vegetable proteins, such as those contained in various kinds of beans, peas, lentils, nuts, and cereals (including oatmeal, milled rice, and wheat), are of poorer quality, or "incomplete" and for this reason need to be supplemented either by one another or by animal protein. There is evidence that it is not satisfactory to have one of the incomplete proteins at one meal and another at a different meal because the amino acids of one food will be "burned" by the body before those which might supplement them from another food are eaten. When reliance must be placed to a great extent on vegetable protein, the practice of serving two or more sources of vegetable protein together is a good one. Grinding cereals and

[3] Unfertilized, "vegetable," eggs may be permitted to Hindus.

legumes together for porridge or bread or serving them together at one meal makes use of whatever supplementary value the two sources may have for one another. The combination of milk with cereal is very good. *Even a small amount of animal protein in the form of milk, cheese, meat, fish, or eggs will supplement relatively large amounts of cereal or legume-seed protein.* Ten per cent of calories should be from protein for an adult and 12 to 15 per cent for a growing child.

Why is it that proteins are so essential to health? It is because, although other food elements can suffice for the production of energy, *nothing but protein can be utilized for building protein parts of the body or replacing protein substances lost in body processes.* The muscles, the organs, the blood, the nervous system, and the gland products are among the body's protein constituents. Antibodies—the substances with which the body fights and conquers disease germs—are also of protein nature. Without the proper amount and quality of protein food the body cannot manufacture antibodies and accordingly may stand a poor chance of recovery from infections. Prospective mothers should have an extra supply of proteins for the needs of the unborn child. Children cannot grow without good proteins in their diet. They need these foods urgently. With deficiency of protein also is associated lack of the important vitamins and minerals contained in protein foods. Famine sufferers deprived entirely of proteins become bloated with dropsy. This is because, when body proteins have become depleted owing to lack of proteins in the diet, water tends to accumulate in the tissues of the body.

Minerals

These, like proteins, are building foods, and they also function in the regulation of body processes.

Calcium is essential for good health and for strong bones and teeth. It is more likely to be deficient in the diet than some other minerals. Vitamin D is essential for the utilization of calcium by the body. Sometimes calcium although present in food, is not well utilized because sunshine (to produce vitamin D in the body) or vitamin D in food is lacking.

Milk is our best source of calcium, and no other food can replace it in that respect. Too much emphasis cannot be placed on the desirability of milk in every diet, but especially in the diet of those in periods of growth: infants and children, pregnant women, nursing mothers. In fact, it is very difficult to plan a diet for a person of any age or condition which meets the standards of the "Recommended Dietary Allowances" for calcium if milk or milk products are not included. But in many areas of the world milk is not available to the majority of the people, and there we must look for other sources of this nutrient.

It is because of the need for calcium and other minerals that animals and human beings sometimes display an appetite for eating clay. The same need explains the habit of gnawing bones. It is said that in parts of Africa where the softer portions of bones are gnawed by the native population the people have excellent teeth. One should be very reluctant to discourage such a practice unless he has something better to offer. Calcium is sometimes added to the diet in various countries by the use of "pot ashes" in cooking, especially the ashes of swamp plants which have been burned, as is the practice in some regions of Africa. Lime is used for making cakes from maize (tortilla) in Mexico, in making bread from rice ("banh duc") in Indo-China, in soybean curd in China, and with the betel leaf and nut in India, Burma, and Malaya. Water used for drinking and cooking may contain lime as well as other mineral salts. Egg shells (calcium carbonate) are sometimes ground up and mixed with cereal when no other source of calcium is available.

In some parts of the world many kinds of small fish, both fresh and dried, are eaten *with all their bones*. The bones supply calcium to many people who have few other sources of the mineral.

In South China an attempt is made to meet the extraordinary need of prospective mothers for calcium by giving them pigs' feet to eat. Sometimes the pigs' feet are cooked in rice vinegar. The slow cooking of bones with an acid will dissolve some of the calcium. It is said that an average serving of spare ribs cooked with vinegar provides an appreciable amount of calcium.

Some varieties of green leaves are among the foods that furnish significant amounts of calcium. In general, green leaves which do *not* have a high content of oxalic acid qualify in this respect. On the other hand spinach (although very valuable in other respects) is, because of its oxalic acid content, one of the greens that are *not* useful as a source of calcium. Malva, however, an uncultivated plant which grows extensively on the Mexican plateau, is an excellent source of calcium. One serving (100 grams), eaten much as we eat spinach, can supply half of the expectant mother's recommended daily supply. Besides calcium malva contains appreciable amounts of iron and vitamins (vitamin A, ascorbic acid, thiamin and niacin).[4]

When sufficient calcium is not present naturally in available food, the mineral may be added in medicinal form. This is well illustrated by the use of calcium lactate or calcium carbonate in preparing milk from soybeans or peanuts in the recipes given in Appendix A. Another illustration of the addition of calcium to food is offered by the following plan which has been used by the Red Cross for feeding famine sufferers in North China. In this case use was made of the purest chalk available.

REFUGEE FEEDING

BREAD:
 60 per cent meal, millet, etc.
 40 per cent peanut meal or soybean meal
SOUP:
 5 gallons water
 4 catties meal (yellow corn contains vitamin A)

---

[4] See the article "Approach to the Nutrition Problems of Other Nations," by Robert S. Harris, *Science,* July 13, 1945.

1 catty pork or vegetable oil (lean pork contains protein and
vitamin B₁)

10 catties fresh vegetable or bean sprouts (allowing beans to
sprout adds vitamin C)

⅕ catty lime stone or chalk (this adds calcium)

⅕ catty salt

(NOTE: The catty of this recipe equals 1⅓ pounds.)

Bone meal, prepared by pounding bones from which all
flesh and fat have been removed, is likewise a good source of
calcium, but it requires proper equipment and considerable
labor to prepare it.

Sometimes a doctor prescribes tablets of some salt of calcium
(see page 257) to supplement the diet for the special needs of
patients such as expectant and nursing mothers. The recommended daily allowance of calcium can be estimated from the
milk requirement under the "Guide for an Adequate Diet"
given earlier in the chapter. The amount of calcium in a quart
of milk has been estimated as 1.159 grams. Thus it would require almost 3 grams of calcium carbonate (chalk) or approximately 9 grams of calcium lactate to furnish calcium equivalent to that in a quart of milk.

Phosphorus. This is another mineral needed by all. The
Food and Nutrition Board has said,

Available evidence indicates that the phosphorus allowances
should be at least equal to those for calcium in the diets of children and of women during the latter part of pregnancy and during
lactation. In the case of other adults the phosphorus allowances
should be approximately 1.5 times those for calcium. In general
it is safe to assume that if the calcium and protein needs are met
through common foods, the phosphorus requirement also will be
covered, because the common foods richest in calcium and protein
are also the best sources of phosphorus.

Iron. Iron is essential in the formation of hemoglobin and
red blood cells which transport oxygen to all the cells of the
body. It is supplied in the diet by liver, egg yolk, spinach,

whole grain cereal, dried fruits, and molasses, among other foods. These are all foods desirable for other reasons besides their content of iron. The Food and Nutrition Board says, "There is evidence that the male adult needs relatively little iron. The need will usually be provided for if the diet is satisfactory in other respects."

Children who are growing, the menstruating woman and the expectant mother have a greater need for iron. In addition, results of experiments suggest that the relative prevalence of iron-deficiency anemias in the tropics, during infancy and childhood, may involve losses of iron in the sweat.

Iron allowances have been deleted from the table of "Recommended Dietary Allowances" given in Appendix A, and iron values are not included in the table of nutritive values, because it is believed that a diet adequate in other respects will be adequate in iron in all normal conditions. When this is not true, it is believed, the condition is pathological and calls for treatment by a clinician.

To compensate for any abnormal loss of blood from the body, as in hemorrhage or when menstruation is too profuse, the doctor usually treats the patient with iron. In malaria, destruction of blood by malaria parasites needs to be compensated for by the use of iron in medicinal form. In hookworm disease large doses of iron together with a diet rich in iron are needed. For those who cannot secure the services of a physician a safe provision in any of these special needs would be the use of one or two 5-grain tablets of ferrous sulfate after each meal. For children a liquid preparation of iron, such as elixir of ferrous sulfate may be employed (see pages 257 and 258).

Iodine. Sea water, seaweed, unrefined salt obtained from the sea, and sea foods all contain iodine, as do the foodstuffs produced in many areas. In other areas, because the soil is deficient or almost totally lacking in iodine, the drinking water of the region, the grains, vegetables, and fruits grown there, and the livestock dependent upon that water and upon locally grown feeds will all be deficient in this element—and so will the people. Because the lack of iodine, especially during the periods of rapid growth, is responsible for the appearance of simple goiter, these regions are known as endemic goiter areas. In such places no locally produced foodstuffs can supply the lack. The Food and Nutrition Board says:

The requirement for iodine is small, probably about 0.002 to 0.004 mg. daily for each kilogram of body weight, or a total of 0.15 to 0.30 mg. daily for the adult. This need is met by the regular use of iodized salt; its use is especially important in adolescence and pregnancy.

Sodium Chloride. Salt is essential for the life of both animals and human beings. It is the only mineral element usually taken separately. As has been mentioned, additional salt is needed to compensate for excessive loss of salt from the body in profuse perspiration. The Food and Nutrition Board reported in 1945:

The need for salt and for water are closely interrelated. A liberal allowance of sodium chloride for the adult is 5 grams daily, except for some persons who sweat profusely. The average normal intake of salt is 10 to 15 grams daily, an amount which meets the salt requirements for a water intake up to 4 liters daily.[5] When sweating is excessive, one additional gram of salt should be consumed for each liter of water in excess of 4 liters daily. With heavy work or in hot climates 20 to 30 grams daily may be consumed with meals and in drinking water. Even then, most persons do not need more salt than usually occurs in prepared foods. It has been shown that after acclimatization people produce sweat that contains only about 1.5 gram to the liter in contrast with a content of 2 to 3 grams for sweat of the unacclimatized person. Consequently after acclimatization, need for increase of salt beyond that of ordinary food disappears.

Fluorine. This mineral, which is present in excess in the drinking water of some localities, giving rise to mottling of tooth enamel, is thought to be useful, in small amounts, for

[5] One gram is about 15 grains. Five grams may be considered to be approximately a heaping teaspoonful. A liter is equal to 1.1 quarts.

preventing tooth decay. Experiments which add exactly the desirable amount of fluorine to the public water supply are now being carried out, and dentists sometimes apply sodium fluoride to the teeth of children.

Copper. According to the Food and Nutrition Board, "The requirement for copper is approximately one-tenth that for iron. A good diet normally will supply sufficient copper."

Other mineral elements are essential to the body, some in considerable quantity, some in very minute amounts, but they will be supplied by any ordinary diet which is adequate in other respects.

Vitamins

Although these substances are found in foods in infinitesimal amounts they cannot be absent from the diet without danger to health, growth, and reproduction. The need for vitamins for prospective and nursing mothers and for children must be emphasized especially. Those most essential to human beings in general are vitamin A, the B-complex vitamins (including thiamin [B_1], nicotinic acid [or niacin, sometimes called the "pellagra-preventive" vitamin], and riboflavin [originally called B_2, or vitamin G]), vitamin C (ascorbic acid), and vitamin D. Vitamin K will be discussed also.

It is the absence of vitamins, together with deficiency of protein, calcium, and in some cases iron, that needs most to be guarded against in the tropics. The summary table of nutritive values of foods in Appendix A will show whether accustomed foods of the reader include the ones required as sources of essential vitamins.

Vitamin A. This vitamin is necessary to the health of the epithelial cells, and to the maintenance of normal conditions of the skin as well as the membranes which line the mouth, nose, and sinuses. It is essential for the ability to see in a dim light, especially after exposure to a bright one. Green and yellow vegetables, which contain a coloring matter called carotene, are useful in producing vitamin A in the body. Accordingly, sweet potatoes, yellow turnips, yellow corn (maize), and other yellow vegetables as well as green ones, have a content of carotene not offered by the white varieties. Yellow corn meal for the same reason is more valuable than white corn meal.

Vitamin A, already formed, is contained in butter, liver and kidney, egg yolk, whole milk, cream, cheese made from whole milk, cod liver oil, halibut liver oil, salmon, and other fish oils. Even the body oils of fish such as salmon contain vitamin A. Pure concentrates of this vitamin may be taken if desired instead of the oil to supplement insufficient sources in the diet (see page 257). Vegetable oils in general make no contribution of vitamin A, with the important exception of the oil of the red palm which is found in some tropical locations.

Vitamin A may be destroyed by long exposure to air, especially at high temperatures; but it is not readily destroyed by ordinary cooking or canning.

The eye diseases xerophthalmia, keratomalacia, night blindness, and a skin condition known as "toad skin" (which has been described as appearing like permanent "goose flesh") may result from a deficiency of vitamin A.

The B-Complex Vitamins. There are many vitamins in this group. Folic acid, used in treatment of certain anemias and of sprue, is one of them. Another, vitamin B_{12}, when given parenterally, is effective in the treatment of sprue and pernicious anemia, and is evidently the anti-pernicious anemia factor of liver. As a group, the B vitamins are related to the health and normal functioning of the gastrointestinal tract. For general purposes of nutrition, the most important of the B vitamins known at the present time are thiamin (or B_1), riboflavin, and nicotinic acid. Ordinary cooking and canning have little effect on these vitamins, although exposure to light rapidly deteriorates riboflavin. Because they are water soluble, they may be lost if cooking water is discarded.

Thiamin (B_1). This is essential to growth; it is important in maintaining a normal appetite and is involved in the metabolism of carbohydrates. Because of the last-named function, the amount of thiamin needed by the body is related to the amount of carbohydrate consumed. Nature has placed a good supply of thiamin in the coating of grains such as rice and wheat; but man often removes this coating by refining processes as in polishing rice and making white flour from wheat. In "enriched" flour thiamin has been added after milling. It is very important to include either whole grains or enriched products in the diet.

Usual sources of thiamin, as will be seen in Appendix A, include, besides whole grains, meat (especially lean pork), dried peas and beans, nuts, green leafy vegetables, tomatoes, milk, egg yolk, and yeast. Thiamin is needed for health and growth by the young and also by adults. It is essential for the efficiency of the digestive and nervous systems. Prospective and nursing mothers have a special need for a larger than usual supply of thiamin. There need be no fear of taking too much thiamin whereas a shortage is, under any circumstances, a serious disadvantage.

The disease beriberi to be described among other vitamin deficiency diseases, occurs in the presence of extreme deficiency of thiamin.

Riboflavin. Riboflavin is involved in the life processes of the cells of practically all active tissues. It promotes growth and general health and is believed to prolong the active life span. Liver, milk, green leaf foods, and lean meats are good sources.

Niacin (or Nicotinic Acid, or Niacin Amide). This is one of the nutrients involved in the prevention and cure of pellagra. Liver and peanut butter are excellent sources of niacin, as are milk, lean meats, eggs, and a variety of green leafy vegetables, especially kale, mustard greens, turnip greens, and collards. While milk does not show a high *content* of niacin, it is of value in the prevention of pellagra. It provides tryptophane, an amino acid which can be changed to niacin in the body, and also is favorable to the multiplication and activity of niacin-forming bacteria in the digestive tract. The allowances for niacin have been deleted from the "Recommended Dietary Allowances" as given in Appendix A and niacin has not been included in the table of nutritive values both because the niacin *content* of a food (as shown by analysis) does not truly represent niacin *value* and also because it is believed that a diet which uses natural food to meet the other allowances will at the same time meet the allowances for niacin.

Ascorbic Acid (or Vitamin C). This substance functions in the formation and maintenance of the intercellular substances, that is, it is essential to the strength of the "cement" between the cells of the tissues of our bodies. Thus it is important in the formation of tooth and bone, in the union of fractured bones, and in wound healing. An acute shortage of this vitamin results in *scurvy*.

In the United States, citrus fruits and tomatoes are chief sources of ascorbic acid, with cabbage and other green vegetables, preferably eaten raw, also furnishing considerable amounts. A glance at the table of nutritive values in Appendix A will show, however, that these are far from being the only important sources of this vitamin. The red haw, used in China, is rich in this substance. The Indian gooseberry, rich in vitamin C, is eaten with benefit by Indian children in spite of its sour taste. Rose hips and black currants are rich sources. Dried fruits will not prevent scurvy although they are useful sources of iron, vitamin A, and B vitamins. Of the fresh fruits oranges, lemons, and grapefruit are better than limes. Fortunately, citrus fruits and tomatoes and their juices can be cooked and canned without the destruction of their vitamin C content. Exposure to air, drying, and long cooking tend to destroy ascorbic acid. It is fairly stable in acid solutions, but is readily destroyed by alkalies. Therefore, baking soda should not be added in cooking if the full ascorbic acid value is to be conserved.

Tender green leaves, such as those of the radish or watercress, contain vitamin C. The diets of some people in India would be more seriously lacking in sources of vitamin C were it not for the pungent and acid condiments such as limes, tamarinds, garlic, and coriander leaves.

Eskimos living on meat exclusively suffer no deficiency of

vitamin C as long as the meat is eaten raw. Where meat is the chief article of diet all parts of the animal may be eaten. The brain, liver, and many other parts of the body have a greater content of vitamin C than has muscle meat. In African races scurvy is common as the result of the destruction of vitamin C by prolonged cooking and steaming of foods.

The bean sprouts which are used in China have been found to be a good source of vitamin C. Peas and pulses can likewise be sprouted for the production of this vitamin.[6]

Uncooked sprouts can be used in salads if the water in which they have been sprouted is known to be safe.

Where natural sources of vitamin C are inadequate the vitamin can be provided in synthetic form as tablets of ascorbic acid (see page 257). In time of sickness a tablet may be dissolved in a fruit drink or in jelly. For infants tablets can be added to bottle feedings. The amount of the vitamin required under various circumstances may be ascertained by reference to the table of recommended dietary allowances.

Vitamin D. Vitamin D is essential for the proper utilization of calcium and phosphorus and so for the normal development of bones and teeth. It is known as the "sunshine vitamin" for it is formed in the body by the action of sunlight on the skin. The intervention of ordinary glass prevents this action but the oiled paper used in windows in certain parts of the Orient transmits a considerable amount of ultraviolet rays.

Most ordinary foods contain only negligible amounts of vitamin D. It is present in abundance, however, in the livers of cod, halibut, and certain other fish. Smaller amounts are found in egg yolk and in the flesh of fat fish, such as salmon.

The Food and Nutrition Board recommends 400 International Units of vitamin D daily for infants and children through adolescence, for women in the latter half of pregnancy, and for nursing mothers (see page 257). As to others, it notes:

[6] For directions see Manson-Bahr, *Manson's Tropical Diseases,* eleventh edition, p. 474.

The need for supplemental vitamin D by vigorous adults leading a normal life seems to be minimum. For persons working at night and for nuns and others whose habits shield them from the sunlight, as well as for elderly persons, the ingestion of small amounts of vitamin D is desirable.

A deficiency of vitamin D may be the cause of *rickets* in children and of *osteomalacia* in adults.

Vitamin K. The Food and Nutrition Board reports:

The requirement for vitamin K usually is satisfied by any good diet except for the infant in utero and for the first few days after birth. Supplemental vitamin K is recommended during the last month of pregnancy. When it has not been given in this manner, it is recommended for the mother preceding delivery or for the baby immediately after birth.

Other Vitamins. There are other known vitamins besides those discussed here. About some of these knowledge is at present inadequate for the evaluation of their significance in the nutrition of human beings. If however, all the vitamins which have been described are made available, there is little likelihood of other important vitamins having been omitted.

Circumstances Which Alter the Nutritional Value of Foods

Vegetable produce may vary in value according to the particular variety or strain, the conditions under which it is grown, and other factors. The vitamin content of milk may change with the food provided the animal. Wilted vegetables and overripe or underripe fruits cannot be expected to be as valuable as foods in perfect condition. For example, spinach which is allowed to stand twenty-four hours at room temperature will lose one-third of its vitamin C. Cabbage which has been chopped will lose its vitamin C rapidly on standing. Overcooking robs foods of vitamins. Accordingly, vegetables should be taken from the fire as soon as they become tender. The minimum amount of water should be used for cooking and whatever liquid remains should not be discarded but utilized in soups, gravies or vegetable "cocktails." Soda should not be added to vegetables since vitamins are more readily destroyed in alkaline solution. Fresh fruits and fruit juices are best consumed as soon as possible after preparation, although the loss of vitamin C from exposure is not so great as was formerly supposed, and it is in any case minimized by keeping the foods cool and covered until use. Milk should not be allowed to stand on the doorstep for a long period after delivery.

Gaining New Knowledge about Nutrition

Many of the indigenous people in tropical countries are healthy and apparently well nourished in spite of comparative poverty as the result of using food substances unknown to the foreigner. Thus gourds eaten as vegetables may not be unpalatable if prepared as they prepare them. Condiments never mentioned in cookbooks, sweets made from milk, kernels of roasted seeds of pumpkin and watermelon and even things which are rather repulsive to the foreigner, as the gray, chalklike dried buttermilk so loved by the Bedouin Arab, may be the determining factor for the absence of deficiency disease. The foreigner should approach such wisdom with respect and willingness to learn. Knowledge which his neighbors can share with him may constitute a contribution to the science of nutrition.

THE QUANTITATIVE ASPECT OF FOOD

IT IS IMPORTANT to know not only *what* food nutrients are needed to *maintain health,* but *how much* of each nutrient is recommended. The Food and Nutrition Board of the National Research Council, Washington, D.C., offers a table which may be used as a yardstick for this purpose. (See Appendix A.)

The measurement of food energy is expressed in terms of calories. The calorie is actually a unit of heat—the amount of heat required to raise the temperature of one kilogram (or 2.2

pounds) of water one degree Centigrade (or 1.8°F.). As they appear in the American diet, each gram of carbohydrate is calculated to furnish to the body the energy equivalent of 4 calories; each gram of protein, 4 calories; each gram of fat, 9 calories. The need of adults for calories, as will be seen in the table of recommended allowances, varies from the 2000 calories recommended for a woman of sedentary habits to the 4500 required by a man doing heavy manual work. In addition to *external* work the body has its *internal* work to do. That is to say, cell activity, the beating of the heart, respiration, digestion of food, the continuance of the muscles in normal tension, etc., must continue even while a person is resting quietly in bed. During illness the presence of fever, delirium or restlessness and losses from the body in discharges, as in diarrhea, give rise to the need for additional calories as well as additional supplies of certain nutrients.

If one consumes more calories than he needs for his degree of activity his body will accumulate fat. There is no other method by which the individual can gain weight. If, on the other hand, he takes fewer calories than are required by his activity, the body will utilize its stored fat to make up the difference, and the body weight will be reduced. There is no other method for reducing.

Desirable Weight

The adult's need for calories is that amount which will maintain his body at the most desirable weight, or bring it to that point if he is above or below it. Tables of desirable weight for men and women, ages twenty-five and over, will be found in Appendix A. These have been prepared by the Statistical Bureau of the Metropolitan Life Insurance Company. Note that account is taken of the body build of the individual: small, medium, or large frame; and that for each type a range of several pounds is given. Within this range probably lies the weight at which each individual of twenty-five years or more will reach his own state of optimum well-being. But note, also, that there is no allowance made for increasing weight with advancing years. The mortality rates of the life insurance companies give proof that such an increase is not desirable. For example, in one study it was found that in men above forty-five years the death rate was 1308 per 100,000 for "normal" weight, but it was 1274 per 100,000 for "underweight" and 1824 for "overweight." Beyond the age of twenty-five or thirty, those who are overweight are more subject than are their lighter brothers and sisters to heart disease, high blood pressure, diabetes, hypoglycemia, disorders of the digestive tract, respiratory diseases, disorders of the bones and joints, and they are much poorer surgical risks—to mention only a few of the possible drawbacks to overweight!

On the other hand, in the years just preceding twenty-five, weight slightly above average is desirable. This is shown, especially, in the mortality rates from tuberculosis and respiratory diseases.

A child needs the number of calories that will keep his body within his own normal range and allow for regular growth. In the past too much emphasis has been laid on an individual child's possible deviation from an "average" weight for his height and age, or an "average" height for his age. It is normal *development* which should be stressed, and height and weight are only two of the criteria of good health. Wetzel has based his chart on these fundamental principles: (1) Healthy progress prefers development along a channel of given body type on an age schedule or timetable specific for the subject and with preservation of that subject's natural physique; and (2) each child should be considered his own standard of comparison.

Weight Reduction

As has been said, the only method by which any person can reduce his body weight is to consume fewer calories than he uses, so that his body's stores of fat will be drawn upon. Overweight is the most prevalent type of malnutrition among American adults today. To say "It runs in my family" is no excuse, for it is probably habits of overeating that are a family trait. Nor should one say, "Everything I eat goes to fat. I use less energy than others do." Only the calories that one eats in excess of his need go to fat, and actually, because he has more weight to move, each move requires more energy than a similar move by a thinner person. Because one is overweight, he probably just does not move so much!

At the same time that the overweight person is reducing the number of calories that he eats, he must not forget that his needed allowances for protein, minerals, and vitamins should be guarded jealously. These needs are in no way decreased. A glance at the table of nutritive values will show that certain foods furnish calories and little besides; these the overweight person cannot afford to eat. Those foods which are low in calories and those which are rich in other nutrients along with their calories are the ones that he will want to use.

A moderate amount of fat in the reducing diet will make it more satisfying and will decrease the likelihood of the individual's becoming hungry before time for the next meal. Three meals a day, some good protein food in each meal, and no between-meal "snacks" should be his schedule. He should guard against the "hidden" calories in the bottle of carbonated beverage, the rich dressing on an otherwise desirable salad, the sauce on his low-calorie fish. Salad dressings made of mineral oil are not desirable, as they rob the body of its fat-soluble vitamins. Short cuts such as appetite depressants and metabolism stimulants are undesirable or dangerous; "reducing ointments" and many other highly advertised nostrums are worthless. Exercise cannot be depended upon for reducing, for it would take one and a half hours of walking at the rate of four miles an hour, or two hours of mowing the lawn (without a power mower!) to use up the energy furnished by a malted milk or by one piece of three-layer cake with icing.

A regular loss of one or two pounds a week is a desirable one for the overweight. This will mean that the diet should contain five hundred to a thousand calories less each day than the body uses. Dr. Mary Swartz Rose used to say, "Don't lose more than two pounds a week, but count that week lost in which you don't lose two pounds."

Increasing Weight

For the *underweight* additional vitamins, and especially thiamin, are useful for improving the appetite. As a rule, however, three generous, well-balanced and attractive meals with plenty of cream and butter included, together with extra nourishment between meals and at bedtime will result in gaining weight. Fruit juices, vegex broth, and "milk-shakes" will supply the need for vitamins. Brewers' yeast powder added to peanut butter makes a nourishing spread for bread and crackers. It is better to get one's vitamins in the natural state as constituents of food whenever possible.

For the underweight, although at least a daily walk out of doors is needed by everyone, it may be well to take less strenuous exercise than has been customary. More than usual sleep and rest is also advisable.

Recommended Allowances for Proteins, Minerals, and Vitamins

Repeated reference has been made in these pages to the Recommended Dietary Allowances of the Food and Nutrition Board. In the words of that board, these are "allowances suitable for maintenance of good nutritional status," and the term "allowances" has been used "to avoid any implication of finality or of minimal or optimal requirements." We have seen that a surplus of food energy calories is not desirable. The allowances for protein, minerals, and vitamins are made to provide for a generous margin of safety.

Not all persons who fail to reach the goal of these allowances will be malnourished; for other persons the allowances may cover only the amounts needed for maintenance. The board says, "The allowances are intended to serve as a guide for planning an adequate diet for every normal person of the population." They are planned for healthy persons of "average" weight, and should be decreased or increased for smaller or larger persons in each category.

They are planned for persons accustomed to American food habits. (Too little is known of the needs of people reared on less liberal diets to be able to say what their allowances should be, but doubtless they could be lower.)

These allowances are for foods as eaten and do not allow for losses in storage, cooking, and serving. Many different patterns in a day's diet and many different types of food may be used to achieve these goals of good nutrition for all.

NUTRITION AT LOW COST

SOME READERS will be responsible for planning the nutrition of large numbers of individuals, as in schools and orphanages, for which they may have a very small appropriation of funds. In such a case, it is well to consider first the nutritive value of the staple food or foods used in the area as sources of food energy. What do these foods contribute? This information probably will be found in part 11 of Table III, in Appendix A, which shows the value of cereals and grain products, starches, and starchy roots. Perhaps, also, there will be soybeans or other legumes, whose nutritive values will be found in parts 8 and 9, or in a few areas there will be oils (part 12) or fruits (as bananas or plantain) among these staple foods. Calculate the nutritive value of these foods in the amounts usually consumed. Then note the total nutrients which are supplied when the food energy needs are met or nearly met. Are there other foods being used in smaller amounts which make a contribution to the total? What might be added to supply the deficiencies? Are there additional foodstuffs which might be used for part of the calory needs that would supply more of other nutrients than do foods now in use? (Be careful of local custom and habit. A diet that may seem deadly monotonous to one who has not been reared on it may be a privilege to be defended to one who has!) But habits *can* be changed in time; new foods can be introduced or, perhaps, appreciation developed for some always available but never appreciated, and so seldom used. Diets *can* be improved within the limits of the budget. Although the goal of good nutrition for the masses may be a long way off, any forward step which can be achieved is well worth the time and effort it costs. In many countries nutritionists and agriculturists working together can give assistance in meeting problems, and they can be helped greatly by folk who belong to neither profession but have good will and an intelligent interest.

PART II

Symptoms and diseases resulting from deficiency of specific vitamins have been mentioned in Part I of this chapter. Few people with seriously inadequate diets have one deficiency alone. Nevertheless certain diseases, due principally to deficiency of one vitamin in particular, present a picture that can be recognized. If recognized, these diseases might be treated successfully by a lay person, in case no medical help is available.

Diseases Due to Deficiencies of the B-Complex Vitamins

Beriberi. This is a disease due principally to the lack of thiamin. It is common among people whose diet consists almost entirely of polished rice from which the coating, containing thiamin together with phosphorus and fat, has been removed in milling. Whether rice is overmilled to the extent of producing danger of berberi can be ascertained by placing a sample in a dish and covering it with Gram's iodine solution. If the entire grain turns black the rice is unsafe for use. Safe rice, being protected by a portion of the external layers, will be only partly stained. In China polishings removed from rice are used as medicine and known as extract of tiki-tiki.

In some places the only item in the native diet capable of preventing beriberi is the fermented drink called "toddy." When this drink is taken away, unless some other source of thiamin is provided, beriberi occurs. One type of beriberi is characterized by paralysis of the lower part of the body so that the patient cannot walk. In the other type the heart is affected with resulting dropsy, giving rise to the term "wet beriberi." "Infantile beriberi" occurs only in breast-fed infants whose mothers subsist on a diet deficient in thiamin. Removal of the infant from the breast and the giving of extract of tiki-tiki results in cure. Untreated infants die in convulsions.

Beriberi can be treated by administering thiamin in pure synthetic form or in combination with other vitamins of the B-complex, as in brewers' yeast. Rice is best eliminated from the diet and less starchy foods used in its place. Beans, peas, peanuts, barley, whole wheat flour and eggs are recommended, supplemented as recovery proceeds by other provision for a well rounded diet. When the heart is involved medical care is imperative.

Pellagra. Pellagra is due chiefly to lack of *nicotinic acid;* but other B-complex vitamins are also needed for its cure. It often, but not always, occurs in populations living chiefly on corn (maize) meal. The use of salt pork does not prevent the disease as do fresh meat, milk and eggs.

Cases range in severity from persons noticing only weakness and a sore tongue and mouth to others suffering from all the other classical symptoms of pellagra, including a skin eruption (like sunburn symmetrically distributed and seen especially on the hands and face), diarrhea, and mental symptoms progressing to dementia. Finally death may ensue, if the condition is untreated.

Treatment consists of administering the B-complex vitamins. Nicotinic acid alone is insufficient; thiamin and riboflavin should also be given. These may be provided in the form of injections of crude liver extract; or by mouth as tablets or capsules of B-Complex vitamins; or in brewers' yeast. Fresh milk, buttermilk, eggs, lean meats, liver and kidney, meat broths, fruit juices and green vegetables should be included in the diet.

Deficiency of Vitamin C (Ascorbic Acid)

Scurvy. This was recognized in former years at it occurred in sailors, cut off, during long journeys in sailing vessels, from all fresh foods. The provision of fresh vegetables was found to prevent it.

Symptoms begin with a feeling of weakness and mental depression accompanied later by painful, bleeding gums and loosened teeth, responsible for a disinclination to eat. The skin becomes rough and dry, is easily bruised and may show small red spots, due to tiny hemorrhages about the roots of hairs. The body becomes painful, as in rheumatism, because of hemorrhage into the muscles. Infants suffering from scurvy, when artificial feeding fails to include the use of fruit juice or ascorbic acid, cry out with pain whenever they are handled.

Profuse hemorrhage from the nose and mouth may precede death from scurvy. These, and other symptoms, are due to abnormal fragility of the blood-vessel walls.

Severe cases of scurvy should be kept in bed and fed with milk and orange juice. Thirty ounces of orange juice daily will result in rapid improvement. Tablets of ascorbic acid in doses of 100 mg. three times a day may be substituted for orange juice. As the gums and teeth become normal, meat, potatoes and fresh vegetables are to be added to the diet.

Deficiency of Vitamin D

Rickets. Evidenced by softening and deformity of bones, this is a disease chiefly affecting infants. Between the ages of four months and two years, symptoms such as bowed legs, "chicken breast," "pot belly," and squareness of the head are recognized. The child is a frail, weak, and poorly developed little sufferer and his head often sweats, wetting the pillow.

Prevention of rickets is best accomplished by giving babies cod liver oil or a vitamin D concentrate such as viosterol or drisdol, together with exposure to sunlight. The less advantage can be taken of sun baths the more urgent is the need for the provision of vitamin D in medicinal form (see page 257).

Treatment. A physician may prescribe large doses of vitamin D. The lay person should confine himself to usual doses. Excessive amounts do harm.

Osteomalacia, or "adult rickets," occurs principally in women who are secluded in harems because of religious custom, with resulting inadequate exposure to sunlight. This disease is seen not infrequently in northern China as well as in India. Deficiency of calcium in the diet is a contributing factor because of the drain of minerals from a mother's body resulting from frequent pregnancies and long-continued breast feeding.

Symptoms in mild cases include pain in the bones of the legs when standing or walking. A "waddling" gait is common. In severe cases great bony deformity occurs, sometimes giving rise to extreme difficulty in childbirth.

Treatment of osteomalacia consists in giving foods rich in calcium and phosphorus, especially milk, cheese, eggs and nuts, supplemented by Vitamin D in medicinal form. Calcium phosphate is beneficial in doses amounting to 3 to 6 drachms (11.6 to 23.2 grams) daily.

SUGGESTED READING

L. Jean Bogert, *Nutrition and Physical Fitness,* fifth edition, W. B. Saunders Company, Philadelphia, 1949.

Margaret S. Chaney and Margaret Ahlborn, *Nutrition,* fourth edition, Houghton Mifflin Company, Boston, 1949.

Adelle Davis, *Vitality Through Planned Nutrition,* revised edition, The Macmillan Company, New York, 1949.

Holger Frederick Kilander, *Nutrition for Health,* McGraw-Hill Book Company, Inc., New York, 1951.

Ruth M. Leverton, *Food Becomes You,* University of Nebraska Press, Lincoln, Nebraska, 1952.

Grace MacLeod and Clara Mae Taylor, *Rose's Foundations of Nutrition,* fourth edition, The Macmillan Company, New York, 1944.

H. H. Mitchell and Majorie Edman, *Nutrition and Climatic Stress,* Charles C. Thomas, Publisher, Springfield, Illinois, 1951 (technical).

Lucius Nicholls, *Tropical Nutrition and Dietetics,* third edition, Bailliere, Tindall & Cox, London, 1951 (technical).

Recommended Daily Dietary Allowances. Revised 1948. National Research Council, (Food and Nutrition Board, Reprint and Circular Series 129) , Washington, D. C., 1948 (technical).

Henry C. Sherman and Caroline S. Lanford, *Essentials of Nutrition,* third edition, The Macmillan Company, New York, 1951.

TABLES OF NUTRITIVE VALUES

Composition of Foods Used in Far Eastern Countries, Agriculture Handbook No. 34, Bureau of Human Nutrition and Home Economics, U. S. Department of Agriculture, 1952.

Composition of Foods—Raw, Processed, Prepared, Agriculture Handbook No. 8, Bureau of Human Nutrition and Home Economics, U. S. Department of Agriculture, 1950.

Food Composition Tables—Recommended for Use in the Philippines, Handbook No. 1, Institute of Nutrition, Department of Health, Republic of the Philippines, 1951.

B. S. Platt, *Tables of Representative Values of Foods Commonly Used in Tropical Countries,* Medical Research Council Special Report Series No. 253, Her Majesty's Stationery Office, London, 1945.

OTHER SOURCES OF HELP

Write to your regional F.A.O. office. If there is none, or if you do not know its address, consult:

Nutrition Division
Food and Agricultural Organization of the United Nations
Viale Terme Di Cavacalla
Rome, Italy

Consult the public health or agricultural authorities of the country or province in which you work. Consult those departments, or those of home economics, nutrition, or biochemistry, in any university in your country or in a neighboring country in which conditions are similar.

U. S. government publications are for sale by the Superintendent of Documents, Washington 25, D. C. (List available upon request.) Free literature on nutrition can be obtained from the Bureau of Human Nutrition and Home Economics, U. S. Department of Agriculture, and from the health departments of the various states in the United States.

Many commercial firms and organizations distribute literature and illustrative material on the subject of nutrition. The following are among those whose material may be considered reliable (usually with special emphasis on the value of the class of foodstuffs to which their own products belong):

The Borden Company, 350 Madison Avenue, New York 17, N.Y.

National Dairy Council, 111 North Canal Street, Chicago 6, Illinois

National Livestock and Meat Board, 407 South Dearborn Street, Chicago 5, Illinois

H. J. Heinz Company, Pittsburgh 12, Pennsylvania

Mead Johnson and Company, Evansville 21, Indiana

Abbott Laboratories, North Chicago, Illinois

Upjohn Company, Kalamazoo, Michigan

11

A FAMILY IN THE TROPICS

PROSPECTIVE PARENTS should supply themselves with literature in the anticipation of successful parenthood, particularly in the tropics where they will be largely dependent on their own resources. The suggestions in this chapter are intended to supplement general information with respect to more special needs in a tropical environment.

All seasons in the tropics are not equally favorable for childbirth, so it is wise to have births coincide with the most comfortable time of year, whenever possible. Even more important is choosing a time for pregnancy when a physician will be available to supervise the expectant mother's condition. Many women enjoy excellent health during pregnancy and can continue many of the usual activities. Certain precautions, however, should be observed.

Strenuous exercise and lifting of heavy objects is forbidden. Inhalation of cleaning fluid and insecticides may have a harmful effect and should be avoided. The use of quinine for malaria may cause abortion, so it is better to use other antimalarials during pregnancy. Malaria itself however is more dangerous during pregnancy than is quinine, so small doses at more frequent intervals may be prescribed when other remedies are unavailable.

The first three months are the period when abortion is most likely to occur. Late hours and fatigue are to be avoided, especially during the days when the menstrual period would ordinarily have occurred. If traveling is unavoidable it should be put off until after the fourth month. There should be no contact with contagious diseases, *especially German measles*.

The health and strength of both mother and child depend largely upon nourishment provided during pregnancy. Extra protein, calcium and vitamins are needed, especially during the latter half of pregnancy. The daily quart of milk recommended may be supplemented by calcium and vitamins in medicinal form, according to the doctor's advice.

Anemia in both mother and child can be prevented by a sufficient quantity of iron. The average need of 12 grams of iron is increased to 15 grams during pregnancy. In regions where goiter is prevalent, iodized salt may be prescribed by the physician.

After the birth of the child, breast feeding is best in any climate, but where milk of good quality is hard to obtain and where germs multiply in it rapidly due to hot weather, it is emphatically desirable. Unless otherwise advised by her physician, the mother should *expect* to nurse her child. Some mothers are disappointed in this respect because of inadequate preparation for breast feeding.

Sore nipples are one reason for failure, and can usually be prevented by care during pregnancy. Nipples should be washed with warm water and soap every night, then massaged with lanolin or other lubricant to prevent cracking at a later date. Application of alcohol once daily during pregnancy is recommended by some doctors. Shape nipples to the baby's mouth by pulling them out and rolling between fingers night and morning. A nipple shield of rubber or plastic (not lead) should be on hand during the first few days of nursing, for sore or retracted nipples. This may be a decisive factor in enabling the mother to nurse her child.

Milk usually fills the breasts the third day after delivery of the child. To insure a sufficient supply throughout the period of nursing, the mother should lead a quiet life, with plenty of rest and no emotional upsets. She will do well to continue a diet rich in proteins, vitamins, calcium and iron. One and a half quarts of milk is the amount recommended for the nursing mother.

Securing breast milk from a woman other than the child's mother may be advised by the physician, particularly in cases where birth is premature. It is urgent that the wet nurse in these cases be given a thorough physical examination, and measures taken to insure her cleanliness. Her own child should also be examined.

Bottle feeding may be necessary, and in any event, a daily "relief bottle" is generally approved after the first month. With this in mind, prospective parents should consult the doctor on infant feeding and make arrangements to secure necessary supplies. Pasteurized goats' or cows' milk may be used but buffalo milk is not suitable for infant feeding.

When supplies of fresh milk are inadequate or of doubtful quality the doctor's choice will often be dried milk or canned evaporated milk. In an emergency for feeding an infant until a doctor can prescribe a formula consult the directions given in appendix A. Directions for preparing soybean milk and peanut milk as a substitute for mother's milk or cow's milk are given on pages 244–246.

The fact that one does become thirsty in hot weather may account for the almost continuous nursing of native babies. A mother who feeds her baby according to schedule must give boiled water to drink between feedings. This need for fluids accounts for some cases of high temperatures in new-born babies.

Supplementary food is required, even by breast-fed infants. With the doctor's approval, concentrates of vitamins A and D should be given daily after the baby's second week. A teaspoonful of orange juice, to furnish vitamin C, diluted with an equal amount of water is usually started between the fourth and sixth week and the amount increased gradually. Instead of this the doctor may prescribe ascorbic acid, dissolved in water or in the bottle feeding. Tomato juice may be used, remembering that its content of vitamin C is half that of equal quantities of orange juice. Juice of the mango has been used successfully for babies and in places where infants are fed with peanut milk or soy bean milk this is often supplemented by plantain water (see page 247). When a baby is constipated an increase in the amount of fruit juice given should have a laxative effect. Prune juice is especially good for this purpose.

Ask the doctor about cereal for the baby. As early as the third month of life special "baby cereals," with vitamins and minerals added, may be used. Native cereals are too coarse to use for infants unless they are cooked for a long time and then put through a sieve. Canned baby foods, vegetables strained or chopped, with or without meat, are excellent but some native vegetables also have been found suitable. "Vegetable marrow" for instance, a vegetable commonly used in the tropics agrees very well with babies. Begin the use of vegetables in the third month by giving two teaspoonfuls of vegetable water, made by mashing such vegetables as spinach or string beans and adding the juice to water, to be given between meals. A fine paste of strained vegetable can be tried in the fourth month. Discontinue foods which seem to disagree.

Egg yolk is almost always available and is a good preventive of anemia. A few babies cannot tolerate it. In most cases a few drops of raw yolk is well borne if added to the bottle feeding (after cooling) when the baby is a few weeks old. Increasing the amount gradually, the baby may in two weeks be getting quarter of a teaspoonful. Two per cent of babies are sensitive to egg yolk and cannot take it. In such cases a little beef juice will serve. Beef steak, ground very fine and cooked a little on a skillet without butter or fat, may be begun in the seventh month. A teaspoonful of this meat, mixed with mashed vegetable, can be tried and if it agrees with the child, given in increasing amounts.

When it is possible, the mother herself should feed the child. Native nurses may not be particular about washing their hands. They have been known to chew the food before putting it into the child's mouth. It is impossible in a book of this kind to give all the needed directions for infant feeding. Such points as have been given are intended principally as a reminder that children should be given all the foods they need. Much of the poor health of children brought up in the tropics in former years was due to inadequate nutrition.

The layette, bassinette and bathing equipment for the infant may safely be of the simplest kind. Scales should be on hand to check the weight from week to week. As the child grows older, the crib will assume considerable importance. It should be equipped with a mosquito net against mosquitoes and flies. A small table and chairs should also be supplied, for early supper before the child is put to bed.

In tropical countries, where smallpox is a common disease, vaccination is needed very early. Immunization should be attempted as early as the tenth day of life or at the end of the first month. When no "take" results, vaccination should be repeated until successful. Other immunizing measures will be used by the physician. Whooping cough vaccine is usually administered in three injections at three-week intervals shortly after the eighth or ninth month of life. At the same time diphtheria toxoid can be injected (three doses at monthly intervals) and immunity tested (Schick test) six months later. Sometimes whooping cough vaccine and diphtheria and tetanus toxoids are injected together. Typhoid vaccine will probably be given not later than the end of the first year.

The three major dangers to foreign children in the tropics are malaria, intestinal diseases and eye infections. The intestinal diseases range from worm infestations, evidenced by vague abdominal pains, to acute or chronic diarrhea or dysentery. In some places round worms are so common that each member of the family has been given a routine weekly dose of worm medicine. This is not advised as a general practice, however.

"Loose bowels" may result from an excess of fat in the milk fed to infants. Chilling of the abdomen and eating of unsuitable foods account for other cases. Foods fried in grease; coarse cereals; fibrous vegetables like corn; nuts and certain fruits such as berries, watermelon and canteloupe are notoriously indigestible for children. Raw apples often cause distress, but scrapings from them are easily digested and are often used in treatment of diarrhea. The texture of pork and veal renders them less suitable than tender beef, lamb and fowl for the young.

Chronic diarrhea may be a result of a deficiency of certain food elements, particularly vitamins of the B-complex. Anemia caused by iron deficiency, may be responsible for diarrhea. The rapid multiplication of bacteria in hot weather requires meticulous sterilization of nursing bottles and kitchen equipment such as meat grinders as well as personal cleanliness in all food handlers. Children should be trained as soon as possible never to drink water or eat food that may be unsafe.

Dysentery is usually recognizable by the presence of blood in loose stools. Diapers soiled by infants suffering from dysentery must not be exposed to flies. Such diapers, preferably made of old muslin, should be burned immediately after use. The danger of a child's becoming infected outside the home must be considered. A definite policy should be formed in the matter of taking children visiting where there is a possibility of unsafe refreshments being served. "Custom" can come to your rescue here. Let it be known from the beginning that it is not your custom to take the children visiting. By setting this policy firmly in the beginning, one avoids risks of offending those whose invitations to the children must be declined.

When traveling with children one should provide safe food and drink for the journey. Some things bought along the way, such as eggs, oranges or bananas, may be safely eaten after being washed and peeled but it is wise not to be entirely dependent on such provisions.

In highly infected malarial regions, triple screening is the practice. Besides the bed net, double screen doors are used at the house entrance. There is usually no reason why children cannot be safely in bed under their nets before the malarial mosquitoes begin to bite in the evening. Many doctors advise regular suppressive doses of anti-malaria drugs.

Eye infections are appallingly prevalent in hot countries. In some places scarcely a family among the native population can be found in which there is not at least one blind eye. Smallpox accounts for many of these casualties, as does trachoma. Flies, fingers and use of contaminated towels spread such infections. In seasons when the flies are very troublesome, many European mothers fasten a chiffon veil, preferably of dark green, around the rim of children's topees. Tied around the neck, this shields the eyes from flies, dust, and sand.

When there is any evidence of infection, a doctor should be consulted immediately.

SUGGESTED READING

Literature on Prenatal Care:

J. Eastman Nicholson, M.D., *Expectant Motherhood,* Little, Brown and Company, Boston.

Carolyn C. Van Blarcom, *Getting Ready to Be a Mother,* revised by Hazel Corbin, The Macmillan Company, New York, 1940.

Hazel Corbin, *Getting Ready to Be a Father,* The Macmillan Company, New York, 1939.

Julius H. Hess, M.D., and Evelyn C. Lundeen, R.N., *The Premature Infant: Its Medical and Nursing Care,* J. B. Lippincott Company, Philadelphia, 1941.

Prenatal Care, Publication No. 4, Children's Bureau, U.S. Department of Labor, Washington, D.C. (price 5 cents).

Note: U.S. government publications are procurable from the Superintendent of Documents, Washington 25, D.C. (list available upon request). They can sometimes be secured free of charge from state health departments.

Literature on Child Care:

Josephine Hemenway Kenyon, M.D., *Healthy Babies Are Happy Babies,* Little, Brown and Company, Boston, 1944.

L. Emmett Holt, Jr., M.D., and Rustin McIntosh, M.D., *Diseases of Infancy and Childhood,* eleventh edition, Appleton-Century-Crofts, Inc., New York, 1940.

Douglas Thom, *Everyday Problems of the Everyday Child,* Appleton-Century-Crofts, Inc., New York, 1927.

Benjamin Spock, M.D., *Baby and Child Care,* Pocket Books, Inc., New York, 1946.

Louise Zabriskie, *Mother and Baby Care in Pictures,* J. B. Lippincott Company, Philadelphia, 1941.

How to Bathe the Baby, Maternity Consultation Service, 1359 York Avenue, New York 21 (price 10 cents).

Food for Children, Farmers' Bulletin No. 1674, U.S. Department of Agriculture, Washington, D.C.

Good Food Habits for Children, Leaflet No. 42, U.S. Department of Agriculture, Washington, D.C.

Publications of the Children's Bureau, U.S. Department of Labor, Washington, D.C.:

Baby's Daily Time Card (price 5 cents a set).
Infant Care, Publication No. 8 (price 10 cents).
The Child from One to Six, Publication No. 30 (price 15 cents).
Child Management, Publication No. 143 (price 10 cents).
Are You Training Your Child to Be Happy? Publication No. 202 (price 10 cents).

WHAT TO DO IN TIMES OF ILLNESS

"CALL THE DOCTOR." That is the instinctive reaction to a serious illness in the home. In many foreign communities, adequate medical service is available. Often physicians from among the nationals are fully qualified, in countries where medical schools teach modern scientific methods. Many a foreigner in the tropics owes his life to a doctor whose color is different from his own.

For the average person living in the tropics there will always be a possibility of securing medical aid. In remote parts, however, one may find himself faced with the choice of employing a witch doctor, a barber with some reputation for medical skill or some other practitioner of strange healing arts. Or he may be able to do something himself in the treatment of family or friends. In some instances the call for a doctor may entail a journey of days or weeks, and someone must "carry on" and care for the patient until the doctor arrives.

Those preparing for foreign service should, when possible, avail themselves of Red Cross courses in First Aid and Home Nursing. A supply of bed linen, a shelf of invalid foods, nursing implements and a medicine kit should be kept on hand for times of illness (see appendix C). It is important that all bottles in the medicine chest be clearly labeled, with instructions for dosage. Drugs should always be kept out of reach of children and preferably under lock and key. The bottle of soothing cough syrup containing a negligible amount of an opiate to the dose may be drained to the last drop by a child or a servant hungry for sweets, with disastrous results.

86

Learning to use a clinical thermometer is important. Reading the mercury level on the sharper edge of this fragile instrument is easily learned. Before taking the temperature, however, the mercury should be shaken down below the 96° mark. A quick snap of the wrist while holding the thermometer firmly at the end opposite to the bulb is sufficient to do this. Before use, the instrument should be washed with cold water, *not* with hot. The reading will be affected, too, if the mouth has been warmed or cooled with food or drink. In very hot weather, when room temperature registers 110 degrees or more, the mercury may continue to rise after the thermometer has been taken from the patient's mouth. Doctors working under such conditions learn to immerse the instrument in cold water immediately before and after use. Cold does not lower the mercury but offsets the effect of the atmosphere.

After use, the part of the thermometer which has been in the mouth should be wiped with cotton or tissue. It should then be washed with soap and water, rinsed under running water and dried before being put away. After use in a contagious illness the instrument should be allowed to stand in alcohol a few minutes before being put away.

The patient should keep the thermometer under the tongue with lips closed for three minutes when the temperature is taken. One can count the pulse for sixty seconds, and the rate of breathing for another minute, then record the findings while waiting. The normal on American thermometers is 98.6°; on English instruments 98.4°—an immaterial difference. On thermometers with the centigrade scale, normal is 37°.

Illness in some individuals is often marked by a rise in temperature; others may be quite ill without fever. A child may develop fever for no apparent reason. Only when the temperature is maintained above the level 99.6° for a considerable time or continues to rise, need a diseased condition be suspected.

When the thermometer cannot be retained under the tongue, as with young children or unconscious persons, temperature may be taken rectally. When no rectal thermometer is available, one of the ordinary variety may be used without injury to delicate tissues if care is taken. In any case the bulb should be well lubricated with vaseline before insertion. The thermometer should be left in the rectum for five minutes. Normal rectal temperature is almost one degree higher than oral temperature and readings must be discounted accordingly.

When there is a rise in temperature, patients should be put to bed. Weakness, severe pain or disability also suggest bed. Both adults and children may object to this measure. With the child one must be firm. Special privileges, such as cutting pictures from old magazines or using favorite crayons, may help in making small patients content with temporary inactivity. Adults may be less tractable, but most reasonable persons will realize that exposure to chill and fatigue may have painful results.

Keeping a feverish patient in bed may prevent spread of infection to others. Most contagious diseases are unrecognizable in the early stages. Measles begins with a feverish cold, and scarlet fever with a sore throat, accompanied by headache, vomiting and a rise in temperature. The danger of contagion is often greatest during the days before diagnosis is made. A separate bedroom is a practical kind of quarantine.

When symptoms are not due to serious infection, they usually subside quickly after the patient has been put to bed. But even after a few days of illness, it is well to continue bed rest for twenty-four hours after the temperature has subsided and continued normal. Activities are to be resumed gradually, with frequent rests until strength returns.

When immediate medical aid is unavailable, the voluntary attendant must try to be both doctor and nurse. With good nursing and simple measures for relief and support, the likelihood of recovery is increased. What can the attendant do for the patient? He can give "expectant treatment," "supportive treatment," and "symptomatic treatment." Sometimes he can administer the "specific treatment," as when anti-malaria medicine is needed for a patient suffering from malaria.

Expectant treatment is given before diagnosis can be made. The patient can be made comfortable as far as possible. Those who have had a course in home nursing enjoy a definite advantage in seeing to this, but even the reading of a textbook on home nursing is very helpful. Anyone who has been a patient himself will remember what a difference good nursing made.

Common sense will remind the attendant to arrange the sickroom conveniently, removing superfluous furniture, arranging for fresh air and sunshine while preventing draught or glare. A sponge bath given in bed, with one part of the body at a time being uncovered, is refreshing after a restless night, as is having the back rubbed with diluted alcohol.

Patients with a high temperature or those who are otherwise very ill should not get out of bed to go to the toilet. A bed pan should be provided, or when this is unnecessary a commode can be placed beside the bed. In any case, chilling and fatigue are to be avoided. When the nurse has other duties than that of caring for the patient, a bell should be placed on the table bedside the patient's bed. A pitcher of water or lemonade with a glass should also be left on the table.

Besides making the patient comfortable, expectant treatment consists of watching for any symptoms that may arise. Trained nurses follow a routine of taking the temperature, pulse, and rate of breathing every four hours, and recording the findings with the day's date and the hours of observation. Notations should be made as to nourishment or medications given, amount of fluid taken, the time of voiding and amount of urine, movements of the bowels, as well as any complaints made by the patient or changes in his condition. If a rash is seen on any part of the body or a cough develops, details concerning the nature and location of the rash, the character of the cough and appearance of sputum should be recorded. It is advisable to keep some sort of written record, particularly if a physician is expected later. Such observations will be of great help to him.

To count the pulse, one places the fingers on the thumb side of the patient's wrist just above the line where it joins the palm. On the outer side of the tendons or "leaders" a throbbing will be felt. These throbs or pulse beats are counted during the course of a minute as measured by the second hand of a watch. The number of respirations per minute is then noted. Keeping fingers on the pulse while watching the rise and fall of the chest or bed clothes will enable one to count the respirations without making the patient self-conscious about his breathing.

The normal pulse rate for the average adult male is about 70 per minute. In women the rate is often nearer 80. The heart of a new-born baby beats about 124 to 144 times a minute. At the age of two the rate varies from 105 to 90 and after that a gradual slowing continues until the adult pulse rate is reached. When there is fever the pulse is usually quickened to the extent of 10 beats for every degree of fever. Thus with four degrees of fever (102.6°), one would expect a man to have a pulse rate of 110. In typhoid fever, however, with a temperature of 103°, the pulse rate may be only 80 or 90.

Temporary quickening of the pulse may result from nervousness or excitement, but a persistently rapid pulse, even without apparent illness, should receive a doctor's attention. Irregularities of rhythm should also be reported. The apparent "skipping" of beats or occasional thumping of the heart in an otherwise normal person, however, may have no greater significance than an indication of fatigue or nervousness.

The rate of breathing when fever is present may be expected to exceed the normal 18 to 20 breaths a minute. In pneumonia, when lungs are greatly congested, respirations may number 30 to 60 per minute. In such a case opening windows or moving the bed to a veranda will provide more oxygen. Propping the patient up in bed may ease breathing.

Infection of the throat may cause fever. This may be tonsillitis or a more diffused inflammation. Inspection can be made by using the handle of a spoon as a tongue depressor. If throat infection is suspected, the examiner should cover his own nose and mouth while making an inspection. Abnormal swelling or redness may be observed in some cases, or perhaps a grayish or whitish membrane or yellowish spots on the tonsils. Mothers should familiarize themselves with the appearance of their children's throats so that changes due to illness can be recognized. Large tonsils are not necessarily diseased. In throat infections, glands the size and shape of beans can often be felt under the skin at the sides of the neck, particularly in cases of German measles.

In cases of nose and throat infection, dishes and silver used by the patient should be sterilized by boiling. Abnormal discharges from the nose, throat and intestines many contain dangerous germs, and should be disinfected. In coughs or throat infections, sputum may be caught on gauze or paper handkerchiefs and burned. Diarrhea, with gradually rising and long continued high temperature, suggests the possibility of typhoid fever and the need for disinfection of sewage. In dysentery and cholera also the need for disinfection is urgent. Every household should have some disinfectant on hand for such purposes.

Eight ounces of crude carbolic acid added to a gallon of water makes an effective disinfectant solution. Other equally good ones are made by adding to a gallon of water 14 ounces of formalin, 3 ounces of cresol or 8 ounces of chlorinated lime. Make sure that the chemical is completely dissolved and that the bottle in which it is stored is tightly corked and labeled POISON. These solutions are to be used full strength only for disinfecting faeces and urine; for other purposes they are to be diluted with two parts of water.

For disinfecting faeces or urine an amount of disinfecting solution equal to the discharges should be added. Hard lumps should be broken up with a stick. Cover the mixture and let it stand for an hour or two before disposal. Patients with typhoid fever or diarrheal diseases should preferably use more than one bed pan. While discharges in one pan are being treated, another will thus be on hand for the patient. Clothing and bed linen soiled by discharges should be soaked for two hours in the disinfecting solution, diluted with two parts of water. They should be boiled before being sent to the laundry.

When emptying the bedpan it is ideal for the attendant to wear rubber gloves, in case the patient is suffering from an intestinal infection. If this is impossible the hands should be scrubbed carefully with soap and water, giving especial attention to the spaces under fingernail, after possible contamination. As an additional precaution the hands may be soaked for a minute after washing in an antiseptic solution. For this purpose one blue tablet of bichloride of mercury, containing about 7 grains may be dissolved in a pint of water; or a teaspoonful of lysol may be added to a pint of water. After the use of lysol the hands should be rinsed in water.

Bichloride of mercury solution must not be used for disinfecting faeces since it does not penetrate solid matter.

A smock or apron, to be donned on entering the sickroom and removed when leaving should hang just inside the room, to prevent spread of infection. When the disease is one against which vaccination is effective, all those who may have been exposed should be revaccinated.

In the absence of a physician, the attendant will need to know how long to isolate the patient. Information as to the incubation period (the time usually elapsing between exposure and first signs of a disease) will enable him to assure himself that others in the household have not contracted the infection. A table of information about communicable diseases is given in appendix B.

When the patient has recovered from a contagious or infectious disease, the sick room must be made safe for occupancy by others. Scrubbing the floor, walls and furniture with soap and water, hanging rugs and blankets in the sunshine will usually be sufficient. After scarlet fever or smallpox bed linen should be boiled. After smallpox, where discharges are very infectious, the mattress and bedding which cannot be boiled or sterilized with steam should be burned. Invalid quarters should be treated with DDT or fumigated with sulphur after diseases conveyed by insects, such as in typhus fever or plague.

Supportive treatment is accomplished by means of nourishment. Starvation or vitamin deficiency usually decreases the likelihood of recovery. In long continued illnesses like typhoid fever, it is a grave mistake to be afraid to feed the patient. Fever increases the need for calories in food. It will not matter seriously if for a day or two nothing but water is accepted or retained, but as soon as the patient can take it appropriate food should be made available to him. While fever is high, nourishment in fluid form is safer; later, as he improves, soft or semisolid foods can be added to the diet. During convalescence, a full but easily digested diet is in order. Not until complete recovery is made should food include other than simple, easily digested dishes. Meals as attractively made up as possible should be served regularly.

The following plans by Rose show how a sufficient number of calories, with all needed food elements, can be given at each stage of illness: [1]

A FLUID DIET FURNISHING 2000 CALORIES

4:00 A.M. 1 cup orange juice with 2 tbsp. lactose (milk sugar)

6   A.M. 1 cup milk

8   A.M. 1 cup gruel: one tbsp. pablum,[2] ¼ cup cream, ½ cup milk

10   A.M. Eggnog: 1 egg, ¾ cup milk, 1 tbsp. lactose, 1 tsp. sugar, vanilla, speck of salt

12   M.   1 cup cream soup: ⅓ cup pea pulp, ⅓ cup cream, ⅓ cup milk.

2   P.M. I cup pineapple juice with 1 tbsp. lactose

4   P.M. Eggnog as at 10 A.M.

6   P.M. Cereal gruel as at 8 A.M.

8   P.M. 1 cup milk

12:00 A.M. Eggnog as at 10 A.M.

A TYPICAL MENU FOR A SOFT OR SEMISOLID DIET FURNISHING 2000–2200 CALORIES

6:00 A.M. 1 cup hot milk (may be flavored with tea or coffee)

8   A.M. ½ cup orange juice
           ⅔ cup cooked farina with added vitamin B_1
           ½ cup thin cream for cereal
           1 thin slice toast with butter

10   A.M. ½ cup orange juice

[1] From Mary Swartz Rose, *Feeding the Family,* fourth edition, pp. 296–299. By permission of The Macmillan Company, publishers.

[2] A specially enriched cereal for infants and invalids. For other foods of this type consult *Accepted Foods,* The American Medical Association (1940).

12   M.   ¾ cup cream soup
 2:30   P.M.   ½ cup prune juice with 1 tbsp. lemon juice and 1 tsp.
                   sugar
 5   P.M.   1 cup hot milk, flavored with tea, coffee or cocoa
                1 thin slice toast with butter
 7   P.M.   ½ cup vegex bouillon
                A one-egg omelet
                1 thin slice toast with butter
                ½ cup junket flavored with cocoa or caramel
10:00   P.M.   1 cup gruel or malted milk
                1 thin slice toast with butter

General Plan for a Convalescent Diet

BREAKFAST   ½ cup orange juice
            Small serving of cereal, either cooked or ready-to-eat
               (giving preference to those with added vitamin B_1
               or adding a small portion of wheat germ)
            ½ cup thin cream for cereal
            A soft-cooked egg
            A thin slice of toast, and butter
            Coffee or tea, half hot milk; or a glass of milk
10:30 A.M. A cup of milk or an eggnog or a glass of fruit juice
LUNCHEON   Meat broth with rice, barley or vermicelli; or cream
               soup (potato, pea, asparagus or tomato)
            Roast or broiled lean meat (beef, chicken, lamb); or
               fish
            Potatoes, baked, boiled or mashed; or macaroni or rice
            Buttered green or yellow vegetable (spinach, carrots,
               peas, asparagus tips) [3]
            Toast, stale bread or plain crackers and butter
            A simple dessert (ice cream, custard, lemon milk sher-
               bet, junket, gelatin jelly, or mild stewed fruit)
            A cup of milk
 3:30 P.M. ½ cup mixed fruit juice (grapefruit and pineapple,
               prune with a little lemon juice, orange and grape-
               fruit); or orange juice
SUPPER   An omelet, soufflé, or small lamb chop
            Toast, or a small baked potato, or rice
            A cup of milk

[3] Small cans of chopped vegetables, offered especially for young children, are excellent for use in invalid feeding.

Stewed or baked fruit (prunes, apples, pears, bananas)
10:00 P.M. A cup of hot malted milk

When a patient expresses a longing for certain foods it is well to comply with his desire unless the food he wishes is thought to be harmful. Ice cream is a favorite and useful form of nourishment for tempting the appetite. When the temperature has become normal a longing for meat can usually be gratified if the following directions given by Bercovitz are followed: [4]

A simple way of preparing meat is to take lean beef and pass it through the meat-chopper twice; then place it in a pan to which has been added a small amount of water. If the chopped meat is stirred into the water as it is being cooked it breaks up into relatively fine granules of meat and the beef extract with the meat granules is finally left. This forms a very palatable base to which boiled rice, macaroni or noodles can be added as desired. Butter to suit the taste may be added.

New foods should be introduced cautiously in the case of a patient who is seriously ill. If diarrhea, a rise in temperature or any other undesirable result follows the experiment of giving a small portion, the offending food should be withdrawn at once.

Until a doctor can be secured, *symptomatic treatment* may be advisable. Even without a diagnosis, something can be done to relieve the patient's distress. Usually the first measure thought of after the patient is in bed, is *giving some form of laxative*. Constipation may be the cause of fever, and in the absence of abdominal pain and tenderness may be relieved by a laxative. Headache from congestion in the sinuses or soreness of the throat is often lessened by free movement of the bowels. Epsom salts, milk of magnesia or other laxatives may be used. *Never use castor oil as a remedy for constipation*. It will move the bowels, and is useful for removal of the irritant in diarrhea or in acute digestive upsets; but its after-effect will be constipation.

[4] Z. Taylor Bercovitz, *Clinical Tropical Medicine* (Paul R. Hober, Inc., Medical Book Department of Harper and Brothers), pp. 562–563.

The following warning should never be forgotten:

In appendicitis, typhoid fever or other conditions of inflammation in the abdomen, it is dangerous to give a laxative. Such action may result in rupture of an abscess or ulcer with resulting peritonitis. Abdominal pain with tenderness and stiffening of muscles over the tender spot when pressure is applied is a positive indication that purging is under no condition to be attempted. When there is no possibility of securing a physician's aid, and it seems really necessary to move the bowels, an enema consisting of one pint of lukewarm water in which a teaspoonful of table salt has been dissolved may be introduced into the rectum slowly by holding the receptacle of water only a few inches above the level of the patient.

When *bloating of the abdomen* is due to the presence of gas and there is no suspicion of appendicitis or other inflammatory process, an enema may be given or turpentine stupes applied to the abdomen. Stupes can be made by sprinkling turpentine on a piece of flannel which has been wrung out of hot water. They should be removed when patient complains of tingling.

Some people have *difficulty in passing urine* while lying on the back. Usually it will do no harm for the patient to sit up. In some cases, water may be trickled into the bedpan over the genitals, thus arousing the impulse to void. In paralytic cases a firm and gentle pressure over the lower part of the abdomen where the bladder is felt to be distended may be effective.

The *relief of pain* may be accomplished in many different ways. Heat has a relaxing effect on tense and painful parts of the body, as in painful menstruation. It speeds the "ripening" of boils and hastens the relief which follows discharge of their contents. Fomentations, made by wringing cloths out in hot water, are excellent, as are electric heating pads and hot water bottles.

Pain which may be due to appendicitis (or other abdominal inflammation) is *not* to be treated by application of heat! It may cause rupture of the appendix. Applied to an abscessed ear, indicated by fever accompanied by earache, heat may have an equally disastrous effect.

Cold may be applied by means of an ice bag or a cool wet

cloth. It is often more effective than heat for the nerve pains of neuralgia or in earache and sometimes serves to retard an inflammatory process.

Aspirin is a useful and relatively safe drug for relief of many kinds of aches and pains. A few people may be unable to take it. If irritation of the stomach follows its administration, a quarter of a teaspoonful of baking soda taken with each dose may help. When this does not remove objections, it is better to desist in trying to use aspirin. The following is a good rule for the untrained nurse: *Never insist on a patient's taking food or medicine to which he believes himself to be peculiarly sensitive.*

Paregoric, a preparation containing a little opium is a useful drug for emergencies. A baby a month old, crying from pain in acute illness, may be given one drop in a little water. At a year of age the dose is 10 drops. Repeat the dose in two hours if necessary. The drug has a constipating effect. It should not, of course, be given in habitual colic.

Tablets containing ½ grain of *codeine sulphate* may be used to ease pain in emergencies for which aspirin is not sufficient. The two drugs may be given together, using two tablets of aspirin and one of codeine. For a child one year old $\frac{1}{20}$ grain of codeine may be used and at four or five years the dose may be $\frac{1}{12}$ to $\frac{1}{6}$ grain.

For the relief of agonizing pain *morphine* is needed. Doctors use it to combat both pain and shock in serious injuries, except in head injuries. If no physician is within call in a community some responsible person should be equipped with morphine in case of emergency.

A tube of hypodermic tablets is a convenient form in which to provide morphine. In these $\frac{1}{6}$ grain of morphine may be combined with $\frac{1}{150}$ grain of atropine sulphate, the latter drug being added to counteract the tendency of morphine to depress the breathing. Hypodermic tablets may be given with a drink of water, as well as by injection.

Only when absolutely necessary should morphine be given to small children. Delicate, poorly nourished infants are especially likely to react unfavorably to the drug. To a strong infant of one year the dose may be ⅓₀ to ¼₄ grain. Although hypodermic tablets are too small to be cut by a knife for division into smaller doses, a tablet can be dissolved in a definite quantity of water, measured in drops, and the resulting solution portioned as desired.

In appendicitis and other inflammatory abdominal conditions morphine given before the arrival of the doctor may "mask the symptoms" and hinder diagnosis. The habit-forming nature of morphine is well known. It should not be used for menstrual pain or other conditions which constantly recur.

Fever indicates the body's response to disease. In some cases it is possible to remove the cause of fever. In malaria, treatment with anti-malaria medicines destroys the malarial organisms and removes the fever. In case of patients who have been exposed to malaria or have had previous attacks it is a good plan to suspect any fever (or even dysentery or apparent heat stroke) of being due to malaria germs. If no doctor can be consulted try giving anti-malaria medicine. If the guess has been correct, symptoms should abate. If not, no harm need be anticipated because of this treatment.

A cool airy place should be selected for the feverish patient, and he should be given copious amounts of cool water to drink. If the temperature taken by mouth reaches 103°, sponge the body with tepid water. This will appreciably lower the fever. Aspirin also may reduce the temperature. If the temperature reaches 105°, wrap the patient in a wet sheet. Keeping the sheet wet, for evaporation, will be more efficient than sponging. If the lips become blue under this treatment, the cold should be removed and the body rubbed with a towel and wrapped in a light blanket.

When *delirium* occurs the patient must be closely watched. To quiet him a dose of 1½ grains of phenobarbital may be given and repeated after 4 hours, if necessary. When delirium cannot be controlled in this way a tablet of morphine may be used.

Faintness or collapse may be treated by giving ½ to 1 teaspoonful of aromatic spirits of ammonia in a little water. Hot tea and coffee are other useful stimulants. Warm covers should be applied.

Vomiting may be an early sign of infection, as in scarlet fever. Do not try to administer food while the stomach is un-retentive. Cracked ice may be held in the mouth at first. Later, sips of ice water may be retained. A mustard plaster applied over the pit of the stomach may decrease nausea and vomiting.

When vomiting is due to indigestible or poisonous food it serves a useful purpose. A dose of castor oil will help rid the stomach of the irritant and will often be followed by cessation of vomiting. It must be remembered however, that vomiting may be a symptom of appendicitis, in which case castor oil must not be given.

Diarrhea is discussed elsewhere on pages 82–83 and 183–184.

Sore throat is a common symptom. Soreness can often be relieved by irrigating the throat with very warm salt solution, using 4 teaspoonfuls of salt to 2 quarts of water. A fountain syringe is used to direct the flow over the inflamed surfaces while the mouth is held over a basin to catch the overflow. The syringe should be sterilized by boiling for 10 minutes before and after use. Aspirin in 5-grain doses, repeated every 4 hours will help give relief. The throat may also be swabbed with 10 per cent argyrol or 1 per cent silver nitrate solution. Inhalation of steam is beneficial when the lining membrane of the throat and bronchial tubes is dry and irritated.

Cough may be treated by various cough medicines, according to the stage of the condition. In the early stages when the cough is dry and "tight" syrup of ipecac is useful. An adult may take 15 drops in water every 3 to 4 hours, or a child of one year, 5 drops. If nausea occurs the dose should be decreased.

For an incessant cough which keeps the patient from resting ¼ to ½ grain of codeine sulfate may be given every 3 hours until relief is obtained.

Pneumonia is not an infrequent cause of death among residents of tropical countries. Cardinal symptoms are a chill, fever, pain in the side, cough and expectoration of "rusty," sticky sputum. Delirium may occur with fever of 104° or higher. These symptoms continue from five to ten days. Then the disease terminates abruptly as a rule. Treatment whenever possible should be specific, with the use of sulfadiazine or penicillin. In general the patient should be kept in bed, protected from exertion and draughts and fed a nourishing liquid diet while fever is high. Administer as much fluid as he will take, especially salty fluids such as clear soup. Three level teaspoonfuls of salt should be taken in 24 hours. When the temperature reaches 103° it should be reduced by sponging.

It is very urgent to secure the services of a doctor who can prescribe specific treatment. Sulfa drugs and penicillin have greatly reduced the mortality from pneumonia.

By *specific treatment* is meant the use of some remedy which is particularly adapted to curing a given disease. Thus atabrine and other anti-malaria drugs are specific for malaria. Fortunately the specifics for malaria are comparatively harmless when properly administered. Sulfa drugs, specific for some of the most dangerous infections, are not so safe. They should never be used when they are not really needed. By one use of these drugs even when applied externally, a patient may be sensitized so that he cannot tolerate them in case of more serious illness at a future date. But sulfa drugs are life-saving remedies in certain kinds of infection. Even the untrained worker would be justified in using them if no doctor can be found for the treatment of desperate illness from pneumonia, blood poisoning, bacillary dysentery or plague. Sulfadiazine is at present the safest of the sulfa drugs.

Doses of sulfadiazine for treatment of bacillary dysentery and of plague are given under the heading of those diseases. For pneumonia, blood poisoning and other very serious infections the following instructions may be followed. The drug is supplied in white tablets containing 0.5 gram (7½ grains). Tablets have a line across the middle to assist in their division. For the use of children the tablet may be cut and crushed and the appropriate dose mixed with syrup.

Doses for adults begin with an initial 4 grams (60 grains or 8 tablets). This is followed by doses of 1 gram (15 grains or 2 tablets) every 4 hours. The medication is continued until the patient has been free from fever for 48 to 72 hours. While taking a sulfa drug a patient should drink enough water to make him void at least 3 pints of urine in 24 hours. It is recommended that he drink 3000 cc. (about 3 quarts) of water during the day and night and a dose of ½ teaspoonful of baking soda three times a day. These precautions are to prevent injury of the kidneys by the drug. Should the urine become bloody or very small in amount the sulfa drug should be discontinued and much fluid given in the form of water, fruit juice, milk, etc. Other possible ill effects, indicating discontinuance of the medication are high fever, a severe body rash, nausea, vomiting, and jaundice. Most patients can take sulfadiazine without ill effects unless they have become sensitized by its administration on a previous occasion.

Dosage of sulfadiazine for *children* may be calculated according to the *weight* of the child. The initial dose should be 45 milligrams (¾ grain) *for each pound of body weight*. After this 60 mg. (1 grain) per pound of body weight per day is to be divided into four to six doses, whichever is most convenient. Thus for a child weighing twenty pounds the first dose would be 1 gram (15 grains or 2 tablets) and after this a dose of 0.25 gram (approximately 4 grains or ½ tablet) would be given five times, at 4-hour intervals, during the rest of the day. Fluid and baking soda should also be administered, in amounts proportionate to the age.

Penicillin is another life-saving drug, useful in serious infections such as pneumonia and blood poisoning. It might be tried in cases which do not respond to sulfadiazine.

As in the case of sulfa drugs, penicillin should not be used unless it is really needed. It also may sensitize a patient so that on a future occasion he will not be able to tolerate the drug. Many preparations of penicillin require refrigeration but forms are now available for which this precaution is not necessary. Directions on the package must be followed in this respect. This drug is often given by injection at intervals of 3 hours. When special preparations are used which are slowly absorbed, one injection into the muscle is sufficient for a period of 24 hours.

"Buffered" tablets for oral use are effective when given in doses four or five times greater than the dose needed by injection. Sometimes a doctor may give one dose by injection and leave instructions for subsequent doses to be administered orally. When given orally the drug should be taken on an empty stomach; i.e., not less than ½ hour before a meal nor less than 1½ hours after eating. Oral tablets usually contain 100,000 units. For pneumonia, for instance, in case no doctor can be secured, two of these tablets, or 200,000 units should be administered as soon as the diagnosis is made. After this, one tablet, or 100,000 units, is to be given approximately every 3 hours, with adjustment to meals, day and night for at least 3 days. This, in successful cases, will usually be at least 48 hours after the patient's temperature has returned to normal.

Doses for children can be calculated in relation to the weight of the child. Considering 150 pounds to be average weight for an adult, a child weighing 75 pounds would be given half the adult dose. For infants the tablets may be dissolved in the formula given.

The use of aspirin should be avoided during administration of penicillin because it may lower temperature and mask the effect of the penicillin. Codeine, however, may be permitted in treatment of cough. Hives are among the unfavorable reactions to penicillin. Sometimes by giving an antihistamine drug such as benadryl or pyribenzamine, the eruption can be controlled so that administration of penicillin can be continued.

Obviously, no specific treatment can be given intelligently until at least a tentative diagnosis has been made. When no medical aid can be secured experienced neighbors may be able to give help in recognizing diseases with which they are familiar. Once the nature of the illness is understood it is not difficult to search a medical textbook for treatments within the scope of the untrained nurse.

In his concern for his patient the attendant must not neglect his own health. He must protect himself not only from disease germs but from fatigue and worry. For the patient's sake he must appear confident and cheerful. In case of failure he must remember that even the most skillful physician with all the resources of modern science cannot save all his patients. He can only do *his* best and "leave the rest."

SUGGESTED READING

Lona L. Trott, R.N., B.S., *American Red Cross Textbook on Home Nursing*, The Blakiston Company, Philadelphia, 1942.

Elinor Norlin and Bessie Donaldson, *Everyday Nursing in the Everyday Home*, The Macmillan Company, New York, 1942.

Lyla M. Ilson, *Improvised Equipment in the Home Care of the Sick*, W. B. Saunders Company, Philadelphia, 1939.

Florence Dakin and Ella M. Thompson, *Simplified Nursing*, J. B. Lippincott Company, Philadelphia, 1941.

L. Jean Bogert and Mame T. Porter, *Dietetics Simplified*, The Macmillan Company, New York, 1940.

Caring for the Sick, John Hancock Mutual Life Insurance Company, Boston (free pamphlet).

Home Care of Communicable Diseases, John Hancock Mutual Life Insurance Company, Boston (free pamphlet).

The Ship's Medicine Chest and First Aid at Sea, Miscellaneous Publication No. 9, U.S. Public Health Service and War Shipping Administration, 1947; for sale by the Superintendent of Documents, Washington 25, D.C.

Harry Beckman, M.D., *Treatment in General Practice*, W. B. Saunders Company, Philadelphia, 1942. (This book is intended for physicians and medical students; it is recommended only for the rare cases of those who must live where medical help is unobtainable.)

Thomas T. Mackie, *Manual of Tropical Medicine*, W. B. Saunders Company, Philadelphia, 1945.

13

COMMON AILMENTS

THE COMMON COLD is too well known to require description. Sufficient rest and sleep, exercise in the open air and a well-balanced diet do much to increase resistance, although nothing has been found which will guarantee immunity.

When fever occurs with a cold, bed rest is imperative to prevent infection spreading to the sinuses, ears and bronchial tubes. The old-fashioned plan of treatment, consisting of a hot bath, a laxative and measures to produce sweating in bed seems to have stood the test of time. Sweating should not be induced unless the patient can stay in bed on the following day. Much water or lemonade should be taken in any case. Dryness in the throat is best treated by inhalation of steam. For a baby the old remedy of rubbing the chest with camphorated oil may be beneficial. A little oil of eucalyptus placed on a handkerchief and left on the pillow near the baby's nose seems to have a good effect. Nose drops of paredrine hydrobromide aqueous may be used to open the air passages of adults or children.

Some young children have frequent attacks of *croup*. This may occur with a cold, or quite without warning. A hoarse cough may waken the parents. The child seems to be in danger of suffocation and it is difficult not to be alarmed. The condition is due to spasm or swelling of the larynx. The morning after the attack all symptoms may have disappeared. Steam inhalations from a regular or improvised croup-kettle may be used effectively. Another remedy is swallowing half a teaspoonful of plain, melted vaseline. Syrup of ipecac is also easily administered. Five drops in a little water may be given to a young baby, or ten drops to a child of two years.

Very often the cause of *headache* is known and can be removed. Eyestrain, constipation, fatigue and malaria are common causes. Migraine is the name given to an extremely painful and incapacitating type of headache, more common in women than in men. It recurs at intervals, affecting the same part of the head consistently. Attacks may coincide with periods of strain or with menstruation.

For relief of severe headache, the patient should go to bed in a quiet darkened room. Hot or cold applications to the head may ease the pain. Aspirin taken in 10-grain doses and repeated every 3 hours when necessary may be helpful. Treatment for malaria may be indicated. A physician will need to study each case of headache individually.

For *earache,* when there is no fever, a hot water bottle may be applied to the ear and a dose of aspirin given. If this is not enough bland warm oil, such as mineral oil, may be dropped into the ear.

When earache is accompanied by fever infection of the middle ear must be suspected. Mastoid abscess causes pain and tenderness in the bony prominence directly behind the ear. Cold should be applied instead of heat in such cases. No time should be lost in consulting a doctor. The use of penicillin or a sulfa drug may prevent the need for operation.

An abscess of the middle ear may rupture spontaneously or the doctor may puncture the ear drum to release the pus. A "running" ear should be kept clean by using a cotton swab wet with boiled water. For a chronic discharge syringe gently with a bulb syringe employing a solution of a teaspoonful of boric acid powder in a cup of warm, boiled water. If the discharge has a foul odor syringe with a solution of potassium permanganate made by dissolving in hot water enough of that chemical to impart a light red color.

The teeth should be checked semiannually or at least annually by a dentist. A good diet and careful cleansing of the teeth do much to prevent decay. In case of *toothache* one must look for a cavity. Food retained in a cavity must first be cleaned out. Then a tiny pledget of absorbent cotton, wet with oil of cloves is to be inserted into the cavity and covered by a bit of dry cotton. Aspirin also will be of benefit.

Menstruation is normally painless. When cramps occur they may be due to faulty hygiene as when fatigue results from keeping late hours or when too little exercise is taken. For some women the taking of a laxative when the flow is expected seems to prevent pain. After pain begins 10 grains of aspirin with a hot drink may be all that is needed. If it is necessary to go to bed a hot water bottle placed over the lower part of the abdomen will be helpful. Recurrent pain should not be tolerated without consulting a doctor.

"Acid indigestion" may be a misleading term. Symptoms thought to arise from indigestion may have their origin in the heart, and vice versa. The periodic "check-up" with the doctor will give an opportunity to investigate the real cause of discomfort. In some cases nervous tension or worry may be at the root of the trouble. This is true also of irritable colon, often wrongly called "colitis."

When excessive acid in the stomach is really the cause of discomfort symptoms are relieved by taking food or alkalis such as baking soda. Such a case may prove to be one of peptic ulcer. If discomfort comes about two hours after meals, when the stomach is empty, try eating a few crackers or a piece of bread, together with a drink of milk if possible. Aluminum hydroxide in either liquid or tablet form will usually give temporary relief at this time. Until a doctor can be found to prescribe for the case diet should be bland and easily digestible, including no fried foods, sour foods, raw fruits or vegetables or highly spiced dishes. Very hot and very cold food or drink should also be avoided. Unless meat is very soft and tender it should be ground; and vegetables containing seeds or fibers such as celery, peas or corn should be put through a sieve before consumption. Rest and relaxation should be provided.

Constipation should be controlled without the habitual use of laxatives. The laxative habit often leads to "irritable colon."

Enemas and laxatives may be used as emergency measures but as a rule the taking of a laxative diet and more exercise than usual can overcome the condition. Mineral oil should not be used day after day since it robs the body of the fat-soluble vitamins contained in food. An abundant supply of laxative foods should be included in the diet. Foods rich in thiamin (B_1) are especially useful. These include wheat germ and dried brewers' yeast or yeast extract. Whole-grain cereals and bread, bran, vegetables rich in celulose such as celery, string beans, lettuce and cabbage are useful and some of these are preferably used raw. Fruit should be eaten liberally at every meal and fruit juices taken frequently. Prunes and other dried fruits, rhubarb, figs, lemons, oranges, tomatoes, and apples usually have a laxative effect as do olive oil, molasses and honey. Water should be drunk freely. A teaspoonful of salt added to a quart of water acts as a laxative.

In discussing the treatment of constipation it should be explained that some perfectly healthy people have a movement of the bowels not oftener than once in two or three days. So long as health is good and no discomfort is felt there is no need for anxiety. On the other hand constipation may be a manifestation of fatigue and treatment may need to be directed to the general condition of the individual.

One should arrange his schedule to allow time for a visit to the bathroom after breakfast or at whatever time the bowels are most likely to move. Many people find that by taking a glass or two of warm water on arising in the morning the problem of constipation is met. A few ounces of orange, lemon or prune juice added to the water increase its effectiveness. A good breakfast should be eaten and all the meals should contain considerable bulk. This is contributed, without unduly increasing calories by including a generous supply of green leaves in the diet.

Hemorrhoids ("piles") consist of dilated veins in the rectum. Bleeding may occur with bowel movements. A doctor should be consulted. For advanced cases surgery is effective. Treatment in the early stages consists in the use of a laxative diet and avoidance of long hours of sitting. After bowel movements any protruding mass should be cleansed, lubricated with vaseline and pushed back into the rectum. Then a short time spent in lying on the right side will decrease congestion. For acute discomfort try sitting in hot water for fifteen or twenty minutes.

Varicose veins usually occur in the leg or groin. Mild cases of distended veins in the leg may be controlled by wearing an elastic stocking or bandage and keeping off the feet as much as possible. For severe cases an operation may be needed.

Neuritis, or inflammation of a nerve may involve one or more nerves. It may be due to disease, such as diabetes or diphtheria or to vitamin deficiency, especially deficiency of thiamin, which often occurs in alcohol addicts. Symptoms include pain along the nerve or numbness and tingling. Until a doctor can be consulted, rest, the application of moist heat, aspirin and a diet rich in thiamin are indicated.

Arthritis, or inflammation of a joint, may be acute or chronic. One variety is a frequent accompaniment of the aging process. The best safeguard against it is good posture and good hygiene, including a well-balanced diet, exercise, plenty of rest and exposure to sunlight. Acute attacks may follow local infections in the teeth, tonsils or other parts. General infections such as gonorrhea and bacillary dysentery may involve the joints.

When fever accompanies swelling of a joint the part should be covered with cotton and put at rest, as when a sling is used for an arm. Medical care is imperative.

Chronic sufferers from painful joints are usually benefited by treatment with heat and massage.

Backache or lumbago. These are often due to faulty posture. Weak arches in the feet may be a contributing cause. A sagging mattress should be replaced by a firm one. The introduction of boards between springs and mattress relieves many cases of backache. Acute cases due to strain from lifting heavy objects or long bending, as in the process of gardening may be recognized. Chairs used for work in the sitting posture need to be regulated in height according to the height of the table used.

Obstinate cases of backache should receive the attention of a physician.

Residents in hot countries are of course subject to many ailments other than those here mentioned. An effort has been made to select some of those in which the sufferer can in a degree ease his own discomfort. It should not be taken as encouragement for the average person to attempt to diagnose and treat his own complaints. Conditions such as cancer or tuberculosis, often curable in the early stages, begin with symptoms unrecognizable except by special tests. Underestimating the importance of "ordinary" symptoms may waste the precious days which hold the only hope of recovery. So have your regular "check-ups" with the doctor and consult him whenever new symptoms arise.

14

MEETING EMERGENCIES

▲▲▲

YOUR FORETHOUGHT in providing a first-aid kit and in studying and keeping handy a *First Aid Text-Book* [1] may be of invaluable help to those about you. If you have actually studied first aid, your assistance will be even more useful. Certainly your success in preventing accidents will have a direct relation to the habitual carefulness you develop in removing potential hazards as soon as they are noticed.

In the study of first aid, one learns that the three kinds of injuries most urgently requiring immediate aid are (1) severe bleeding, (2) cessation of breathing and (3) poisoning. Even when the doctor arrives within fifteen minutes after the accident, he may be too late in such cases unless first aid has been administered. You should completely familiarize yourself with the Red Cross *First Aid Text-Book* to meet common emergencies. Additional treatment that may be given for specific emergencies is suggested below in this chapter.

Fractures. Follow treatment recommended in the first-aid handbook. The pioneer in remoter sections may have to care for a broken arm or leg for a considerable period before a doctor can be secured. Routine first aid instruction does not prepare him for this. When pain is severe the first step is perhaps to give the patient a dose of ⅙ grain of morphine. Then the injured limb is to be gotten into as nearly normal shape as possible by applying traction as described in the first-aid hand-

[1] American Red Cross, *First Aid Text-Book,* revised edition (The Blakiston Company, Philadelphia, Pennsylvania).

book. If it is at all possible to secure medical help, broken bones which protrude should not be made to return to their normal place by anyone but a doctor. Penicillin or sulfa drugs are used to *prevent* infection in a compound fracture.

In fractures of the thigh, the traction splint could be used continuously in case no medical care could be secured. But with this kind of splint there is even more need than usual for watching that the splint does not bind too tightly and irritate the part. Blueness and coldness of toes and fingers mean that the circulation of a part is suffering and that bandages must be loosened.

Dressings on fractures should be changed every three or four days, or oftener if bandages become loose or give rise to discomfort. With each change, the skin should be bathed with alcohol, and any reddened parts powdered with borated talcum and more efficiently padded. While the splint is temporarily removed, assistants should exert a steady pull on the limb to keep it "on the stretch." After the tenth day, gentle massage of muscles about the fracture should be begun. During the third week, the doctor begins *passive motion* to neighboring joints, moving joints such as the knee or elbow gradually without effort on the patient's part. These movements are slowly increased until joints move freely. Massage and passive motion should be continued daily from the third week until two weeks after splint is removed. Most fractures heal completely within six weeks.

Heat Exhaustion, Heatstroke or Sunstroke, and Heat Cramps. Follow treatment recommended in the first-aid handbook. *Heat exhaustion* is not a dangerous condition and is easily treated by having the patient lie down in a comfortable place, covering him if he feels chilly, and giving him a stimulant such as aromatic spirits of ammonia or hot tea or coffee and also a tablespoonful of salt, a little at a time. *Heat stroke* and *sunstroke,* on the other hand, are often fatal. The body temperature may rise to 107° or even 110° and unconsciousness become so complete that the patient cannot be roused. It is very urgent to lower the temperature, by wrapping the patient in a sheet on which cold water is poured, applying ice bags to the head and other parts of the body, placing the patient in a cool bath to which ice is added, or even giving an enema of ice water. When rectal temperature falls below 103°, cold should be removed, to be returned if the fever mounts again. Weakening of the pulse and blueness of the lips and face indicate that cold applications should be removed. In such a case the limbs should be rubbed toward the heart and the body wrapped in a light, dry blanket. Before the patient becomes unconscious he may be given salt with water, as in heat exhaustion.

Burns. Follow treatment recommended in the first-aid handbook. Deep burns produce scars, and scar tissue always tends to contract. As a result, deep burns on the inner side of joints are almost always sure to cause deformity unless a splint is applied, to keep the part extended. Thus on the palm surface of the hands or fingers, on the under side of the knee or the inside of the elbow joint, a splint should be placed over the dressing.

Wounds. Follow treatment recommended in the first-aid handbook. When a doctor cannot be secured at once, apply tincture of zephiran or 2 per cent tincture of iodine to the wound. Apply a sterile dressing after this has dried. Sterile dressings must always be ready for times of need.

Several methods of *home-sterilization* are effective. Packages of dressings, wrapped in muslin, may be sterilized for an hour in a pressure cooker. Or they may be placed with a potato in a hot oven and left until the potato is done. In an emergency clean muslin may be used after being scorched with a hot iron.

In serious wounds and burns most doctors now give penicillin or sulfa drugs to *prevent* infection. This, together with intravenous injection of plasma or transfusion of blood, is often the measure on which life depends.

Dangerous germs entering wounds or taken into the uterus at time of childbirth may get into the blood in overwhelming numbers, causing *septicemia,* or *"blood poisoning."* This gives rise to chills, high irregular fever and drenching sweats. Since malaria causes these same symptoms an attack of malaria, occuring after an operation or childbirth is sometimes mistaken for blood poisoning. Treatment for malaria would cause symptoms to disappear in such a case. In blood poisoning and in serious local infections penicillin and sulfa drugs save many lives.

Boils and carbuncles. These result from infection entering the skin where its resistance is impaired, as from the friction of a stiff collar or by constant sweating. After a long period of hot weather it is common for people to suffer from crops of boils. Pus from one boil may soil the clothing and give rise to new infections. Carbuncles are more extensive than boils. In them pus finally exudes from several openings.

Penicillin, administered at an early stage may cut short the course of a boil or carbuncle, or even a breast abscess, but it is not effective applied in dressings, locally.

First-aid treatment of local infection, whether resulting from wounds or in the form of boils, carbuncles, or abscesses of various kinds, consists in applying moist heat. Six heaping tablespoons of Epsom salt or three heaping tablespoons of salt are dissolved in a quart of hot water. This may be used for soaking an infected hand or foot for an hour at a time, at intervals of three hours. The water should be kept as warm as can be borne. In other cases it will be more convenient to apply compresses, such as a bath towel wrung out of the hot solution, and covered by a hot water bottle. Keeping the part elevated will relieve the pain. This treatment with moist heat will not only ease suffering but will serve to "ripen" a boil or abscess so that it will be ready for operation when a doctor finally arrives. Or a boil may rupture spontaneously after this treatment.

Boils should never be squeezed. To do so may force infection through the protective capsule which nature provides, into surrounding tissues. When a boil has burst, cotton wet in alcohol may be used to gently stroke the swelling toward the opening and assist in removal of pus. Bathing of the skin surrounding the infection with alcohol on clean cotton may prevent the formation of new boils. A sterile dressing should be applied to the infection at least once daily. Finally the capsule, sometimes called the core of the boil will be discharged. After that healing will take place quickly.

The hands of the person who treats an infection of this kind must be washed very thoroughly with soap and water, both before and after treatment. Preferably, sterile rubber gloves should be worn. All cotton and dressings soiled with discharges should be burned.

The surgical opening of a boil or an abscess may be indicated when pain is great or fever present. It should not be attempted until one is sure that pus is present. If this is the case one part of the swelling is usually more prominent than the rest, and by pressing here with the fingers the liquid contents within are felt to fluctuate. The surface is usually reddened, shiny, and hot to the touch. Only a surgeon should undertake the incision of a deep abscess on the sides of the front of the neck, or in the arm pit, the groin or other locations where large blood vessels are present.

The skin, before an operation, should be washed with soap and water and then painted with an antiseptic. Any instruments to be used should be boiled for ten minutes. Unless dry sterile gauze is available, boil squares of muslin with the instruments. These are for sponging and later for covering the wound. Then carefully pour off the water, leaving the other contents of the pan untouched on its sterile surface. Sterile instruments must not be touched until the operator has scrubbed his hands. Sterile dressings should be made ready for use after the operation.

If rubber gloves are available for the operator these should be wrapped in muslin and weighted down to keep them from floating on the surface of the water in which they are boiled for ten minutes. In any case the operator should scrub his hands very thoroughly with soap and water and a brush which has been boiled. Finger nails should be pared and the spaces under them carefully cleansed before the scrubbing. If blue tablets of bichloride of mercury are available a solution of one tablet in a pint of water may be used for soaking the hands after the scrubbing.

On the extremities, particularly in fingers and toes, an incision should be made longitudinally, rather than across the part. In a breast abscess the cut should radiate from the nipple, to avoid cutting across milk ducts.

Rabies, or hydrophobia. Follow treatment recommended in

the first-aid handbook. If rabies is suspected, the wound should be cauterized with pure carbolic acid, followed immediately by 95 per cent alcohol to prevent burning. Find out in advance where the nearest facilities for receiving Pasteur treatment are located so that you will be ready in time of need. Remember that in bites on the face or when the animal suspected of being rabid cannot be examined, Pasteur treatment should be given at once.

Snake Bite. Poisonous snakes are common in some parts of the tropics but their bites are not met with so frequently as might be expected. As a rule snakes bite only when startled and in self-defense.

Those living in snake-infested regions should never put a hand or foot into a place not clearly seen. Use a searchlight or lantern at night, and inspect shoes before you put them on. Keep grounds around residences clear of underbrush which might harbor snakes, and rid the premises of rats and mice, which are a dietary delicacy for them. Wear leather boots or puttees when walking through underbrush.

Antivenin, appropriate for snakes of the region should be kept on hand by the doctor or some other responsible member of the community. In liquid form antivenin requires refrigeration, but dehydrated products will keep at room temperature. Snake bite kits are available, with complete instructions for use of the equipment they contain.

The bite of a poisonous snake, unlike that of a harmless reptile, leaves two puncture marks, unless one fang has failed to enter the skin. The effect of the venom depends on the variety of snake, but in general the poisonous action is on either the nerves or the blood. In the former case general symptoms predominate and death may result from failing respiration, from within an hour to six days after the bite. When the action is on the blood, violent local reaction occurs, with severe pain, swelling, hemorrhage and sometimes gangrene of the part. In fatal cases of this variety death often occurs after six to twelve hours. Some venoms have both actions.

Follow treatment recommended in the first-aid handbook. If no regular or improvised suction cup is available, the mouth may be used, provided there is no break in its lining membrane. If possible, the mouth should be washed out afterward with water in which enough potassium permanganate has been dissolved to impart a light red color. The old-fashioned treatments of rubbing potassium permanganate crystals into the wound or giving the patient whiskey to drink are *not* advised.

When a person is bitten by a snake, the reptile should be killed and examined as soon as possible to ascertain what kind of antivenin is needed. Examination must be cautious since a snake may bite reflexively after death. The appropriate antivenin should be injected at the earliest possible moment. Three to five ampules injected into the swelling around the bite, with several more injected above the tourniquet, may be sufficient. Children require larger doses than adults. If the patient is getting worse, a few more injections may be given.

Insect Bites. In general, these are to be treated by the application of an alkali, such as baking soda or ammonia water. When suffering is great a teaspoonful of baking soda may be given internally. A bee or wasp may leave its sting in the flesh of the victim. If this is seen it should be extracted with sterile tweezers.

Scorpion Bites. These sometimes induce nausea and vomiting, sweating and drowsiness, as well as local burning pain; or simply pain may be the only complaint. In some extreme cases death may ensue, but victims who survive for three hours usually recover. The danger is greatest in the case of infants. During the day scorpions lie hidden beneath stones, buildings, lumber piles, and other sheltering objects. In houses they may hide in shoes or clothing. Fumigation with sulphur is effective against them in the home.

Treatment begins with application of a drop of strong ammonia to the bite, followed by application of a constricting bandage, incision and suction as in snake bite. In extreme cases where breathing begins to fail, artificial respiration should be performed.

The black widow spider's bite is so painful that a dose of morphine is justified. A doctor may inject 10 cc. of 10 per cent calcium gluconate, intravenously. Painful parts may be relieved by application of hot, wet packs. This spider, of a shining black hue with reddish marks on the underside of its abdomen, is found under logs and bridges, in cellars and especially under privy seats. Spraying under seats with creosote is recommended as a preventive measure.

WHEN THE BABY ARRIVES
BEFORE THE DOCTOR

THIS CHAPTER is written for the sake of any person who might have thrust upon him the responsibility of caring for a woman in childbirth. Although normally, provisions for the coming of a child are made well in advance, with medical care and even hospitalization provided for, our best laid plans can still "gang agley" in such fashion that these services are unavailable at a crucial time.

Many animals care for themselves when their young are born. Nature, having started to bring an infant into the world, is very likely to complete the process, either with or without human assistance. A person with some knowledge of the fundamentals can give a great deal of help. The attendant can comfort himself with this thought, then go ahead and do his best.

If the prospective mother has borne children, she will know what to expect. Otherwise she should be told that cramping pains in the back and lower abdomen at regular intervals are likely to occur for a good many hours. These pains, slight and infrequent in the beginning of labor, gradually increase in severity and frequency, becoming almost continuous just before the child is born. The patient may walk about and assist in preparations for the birth until the pains become hard to bear. Then she should have an enema, followed by a warm sponge bath, and recline on the bed.

If the patient's pains are severe and close together at the

time of the attendant's arrival, he should at once begin sterilizing the most urgently needed supplies. Foremost among these are scissors for severing the umbilical cord and four pieces of tape, narrow gauze bandage or strips of clean cloth about six inches long, for tying the cord. These should be placed in a pan of water and boiled for ten minutes. Sterile gauze "sponges" will also be needed and if none are available a dozen six-inch squares of clean muslin may be boiled with the other supplies. Other provisions must be made for the attendant to wash and disinfect his hands. Two basins, soap and a clean nail brush will be needed. In one basin an antiseptic solution may be prepared for soaking the hands after they have been scrubbed in the other basin with soap and water. The mattress on the bed should be protected by a rubber sheet or other waterproof material, beneath the bottom sheet. During the birth of the child some sort of large pads will be needed as further protection. Sterile sanitary napkins will also be required for the mother's use after the birth. In an emergency any soft, clean material may be used.

The first stage of labor is that in which the patient is usually able to walk about. This stage may last fifteen hours. In extremely quick labors the child is born a few minutes after the beginning of pains. Pains in the first stage are due to the dilating of the mouth of the uterus. In the course of dilation some blood tinged mucus is discharged, and there is likely to be a sudden gush of clear fluid when dilation is complete.

The second stage begins with the flood of clear fluid, and is also marked by a tendency on the mother's part to bear down, as in the act of straining during a difficult bowel movement. This stage should be spent in bed. Contractions are now more frequent and painful, having for their purpose the expulsion of the child. The mother can help achieve this by bearing down. She should lie on her back with knees up and brace her feet against the bed. She may pull on a sheet tied to the foot of the bed. Between pains she should rest.

A child is normally born head first. The attendant will need to watch the progress of the descending head of the child. As pains increase in severity and frequency a bulging of the parts before the child's head will be observed. Soon the lips of the genitals separate and the scalp of the infant appears between them. The attendant, having scrubbed his hands with soap and water and soaked them for a few minutes in the antiseptic solution, should have assistance at this point, so that he need not touch anything except the sterile dressings and, in time, the baby and its cord.

It is better that the head should not be born too precipitately. Sitting at the side of the bed, the attendant can hold the head back when birth is imminent, by pressing upward against the baby's scalp at the height of each pain, using a sterile compress. Another compress should be used to support and reinforce by pressure the thinning layer of flesh in front of the mother's rectum, to prevent tearing of the tissues.

Finally the head will be entirely expelled. The umbilical cord (the cord attached to the baby's navel) is sometimes wrapped about the child's neck. It is bluish in color and about as thick as a finger. It can be loosened with the fingers and slipped over the baby's head. When wound so tightly that it cannot be moved, it must be tied at once with pieces of the sterile tape, in two places several inches apart, then cut with the sterile scissors between the tapes to prevent its strangling the infant. One or more pains after this will probably result in expulsion of the entire body. The child, received into the hands of the attendant, will then be wrapped in a sterile towel, which has been warmed if the room is cold, or in a piece of cotton flannel prepared for the purpose.

Immediately after birth, the baby should be held upside down by the ankles, with one of the attendant's fingers between the feet to prevent slipping. The umbilical cord should not become taut during this process. While the infant is upside down, the head should be bent back and the mouth wiped out with sterile gauze. If the baby has not yet cried, the skin over his spine should be rubbed briskly with a towel. If breathing is still not evident, his body should be immersed in a basin of water which, tested by elbow, feels warmer than the elbow, but not hot.

After the baby has cried, lay him between the mother's legs

for the tying of the cord. This is usually done about five minutes after birth or when the cord has ceased to pulsate. One
piece of tape is tied tightly about the cord two inches from
the baby's navel, using a square knot. A second piece is tied
about two inches farther from the child. The cord is then cut
between the tapes, using sterile scissors. If either of the cut
ends continues to bleed, it should be tied again with another
piece of tape. Apply a sterile dressing surrounding the stump
of the cord on the baby and keep it in place with a band about
the child's abdomen.

At this point, if the mother is not in pain, drops may be put
into the baby's eyes. Infection of eyes sometimes occurs during
the descent through the birth canal. First wash the eyes with
boric acid lotion. Then one drop of 1 per cent solution of silver
nitrate is dropped into each eye. As soon as this is done, the
eyes are to be *washed out again,* using several drops of "normal" salt solution (1 teaspoonful of table salt to an 8-ounce
water glass of boiled water). Then wash out with boric lotion
again. After this care the baby may be put into his bed and his
body covered. From time to time someone should observe him
to see that breathing is normal and that there is no bleeding
from the navel.

The third stage of labor is still to be accomplished after the
baby's birth. The placenta, commonly called the "afterbirth"
must be expelled. This is a large, flat, fleshy mass with the umbilical cord emerging from near its center and the remnants
of the membranous sac attached at its circumference. It is often
delivered as the result of one contraction of the uterus, soon
after the birth of the child. The third stage is usually over
within a half hour, but even should it be necessary to wait
much longer, one must *never pull on the umbilical cord* in an
effort to hasten its expulsion. Keep the mother warm, reassure
her, and massage the uterus, exerting firm downward pressure
through the abdominal wall. Unless a doctor is expected, the
placenta may be taken away and buried upon completion of
the third stage. A doctor would wish to have the placenta kept
for his inspection.

After expulsion of the placenta the uterus should contract

so that it feels like a hard ball below the level of the mother's navel. In the absence of normal contraction it will feel soft and flabby, a condition predisposing to hemorrhage. To prevent excess bleeding, press gently on the uterus through the abdominal wall to encourage the uterine muscle to contract. A normal amount of bleeding can be expected but when blood pours out in a flood the foot of the bed should be elevated higher than the head and a teaspoonful of fluid extract of ergot, diluted with water be given the patient to drink. Ergot, however, should *not* be administered before the afterbirth has been expelled.

When the birth is safely over, the patient and her bed are to be cleaned up. The skin, where soiled, should be washed with boiled water. A sanitary pad is put in place to receive discharge from the uterus. A folded towel pressing on the top of the uterus through the abdominal wall is held in place by a broad abdominal binder. When soiled sheets and nightgown have been replaced, the mother should be covered warmly, given a warm drink and allowed to sleep. The sanitary pad is to be inspected occasionally, and another teaspoonful of the ergot extract given if bleeding continues too freely. During convalescence the sanitary pad is to be changed frequently and external genitals kept clean by washing with boiled water.

Aftercare of the child is undertaken when the mother's welfare has been assured. Some babies at birth are covered with a cheesy material, called the "vernix caseosa." In many maternity hospitals this is not removed since the child may derive benefit from the coating. If the child is soiled with blood, the area involved is cleansed with sterile mineral oil or vegetable oil.

If the baby is bathed soon after birth, the stump of the umbilical cord should not come into contact with the water. Sprinkled with boric acid powder, it should be surrounded by dry sterile gauze to prevent its surface from touching the abdominal skin. The dressing is changed daily and a band is needed to keep it in place. When kept dry and uninfected, the cord will drop off after a week, leaving a healthy navel.

In feeding the child, warm boiled water should be given

every two hours. A nursing bottle, medicine dropper or tea-spoon may be employed, after sterilization. When the baby is twelve hours old, he is customarily put to the mother's breast for five minutes. This is repeated at eighteen and twenty-four hours. At the end of twenty-four hours the child is put on a three-hour nursing schedule, with water given between feed-ings. Milk should fill the mother's breasts on the third day.

The mother's convalescence should begin with at least a week, spent mostly in bed. After the first day if she feels well she may go to a near-by toilet, rather than using a bedpan. In bed, she should exercise her legs, bending and stretching them frequently to favor good circulation. She may sit in a chair oc-casionally and on the seventh day begin to walk about for short periods, taking care to avoid fatigue. For several months she must be careful not to lift heavy weights, thus stretching weak-ened ligaments. She should make it a rule to empty the bladder every two hours and avoid lying on the back when the bladder is full.

Signs of miscarriage during pregnancy—recurring pains in the lower abdomen or back, with perhaps bleeding from the uterus—are an indication that a doctor must be called at once. Put the patient to bed. Avoid giving laxatives or quinine.

After a miscarriage, before another pregnancy occurs, a physician should study the case to discover the reason for loss of the child and take measures to prevent a repetition.

Whenever a child is born to foreign parents in an out-of-the-way place where there is no doctor to furnish a birth certificate, the person who assists in the birth should sign a written statement about the birth. This should be registered at the nearest consulate or embassy of the parents' nationality at the earliest possible date.

SUGGESTED READING

Anita Jones, *A Manual for Teaching Midwives,* Publication No. 260, Children's Bureau, U.S. Department of Labor, Washing-ton, D.C.

Henry L. Woodward and Bernice Gardner, *Obstetric Management and Nursing,* F. A. Davis Company, Philadelphia, 1940.

DISEASES OF THE SKIN

SKIN DISEASES are common in the tropics. But soap and water cleanliness; protection from insects through screening; the wearing of shoes and adequate nutrition do much to prevent these diseases. Contact with persons and animals suffering from skin eruptions is to be avoided, as the sharing of towels with any persons at all. Borrowing of slippers, bathing suits, etc. may be the means of contracting a skin disease.

Insect bites, contact with poisonous or irritating substances, such as poison ivy or certain Oriental lacquers and sensitivity, or allergy of the individual to certain foods, drugs, fabrics, etc., may result in uncomfortable skin conditions. Use of DDT or other insecticides and repellents should suffice for control of insects, while in cases of contact with an irritant, such as poison ivy, the affected parts must be cleansed thoroughly with soap and water and a soothing lotion applied. When eruptions are due to sensitivity elimination of the offending substance automatically cures the disease. For temporary relief of discomfort from allergy the anti-histamine drugs, such as Benadryl and Pyribenzamine are a great boon, particularly in the skin eruption known as "hives."

In *hives* (urticaria or nettlerash) the eruption often resembles mosquito bites, running together to form large, swollen blotches in which itching and burning are intense. The eruption may vanish after an hour or two, leaving no traces, only to reappear in the same or some other part of the body. In many cases the attack is caused by some food which has been eaten. Sea food, canned goods, pork, corn and tomatoes are common offenders. Treatment should begin with a dose of Epsom salt to clear the digestive tract. After this, the diet should be liquid at first, with soft foods permitted later. As a relief for local itching and burning, cold compresses of a solution of baking soda may be tried. Calamine lotion (with addition of 5 grains of carbolic acid to the ounce) may also be effective. But this should not be used on moist or hairy surfaces. Starch baths (1 cup of cornstarch in cold water added to the bath) may help.

Prickly heat, characterized by a fine, reddish rash and minute shiny blisters, and accompanied by unbearable pricking and itching, is the result of almost continuous perspiration. The irritation may be due to the presence of a fungus which invades the skin when its resistance is broken down by sweating. The use of soap should be discontinued in such a case, since it increases irritation. Strenuous exercise, hot drinks or anything which increases perspiration should be avoided as much as possible. Borated talcum powder or a dusting powder of equal parts of zinc oxide, boric acid and starch should be used frequently. Calamine lotion patted on the parts and allowed to dry, may give relief. For destroying the fungus diluted vinegar or a lotion of potassium permanganate may be used. Sufferers from severe cases should have a vacation from a humid climate or at least, provision for sleeping in an airconditioned room. This will cause prickly heat to disappear over night.

Acne of a very severe, "cystic" type occurs in some parts of the tropics. In this form pimples develop into cysts, filled with fluid. As in other forms of acne, general measures for treatment include adherence to a simple diet, eliminating chocolate, nuts and greasy foods, and the application of sulphur in some form, such as sulphur ointment, until the skin begins to peel. Cysts should be opened surgically. In extreme cases of cystic acne a change of climate is imperative.

Ringworm, due to a number of varieties of fungus infection, is not infrequent in the tropics. *Athlete's foot,* perhaps the most common, is caused by a fungus which thrives in the warmth and dampness between toes. Floors of public bathing places and showers are particularly dangerous as sources of infection. Bathing slippers should be kept on the feet in both places and should be dried, aired in the sun and powdered before the next use. Spaces between toes must always be dried thoroughly and preferably powdered. "Desenex" powder is particularly effective both in prevention and cure of athlete's foot. Irritating ointments, such as Whitfield's ointment are suitable only for unirritated, dry conditions of scaling and cracking between the toes. They should be applied after washing and drying the feet at night and washed off in the morning. Then after thorough drying, powder should be applied. After each week of treatment with ointment, powder alone should be used for the succeeding week.

For acutely irritated cases of athlete's foot the best treatment is that of soaking the feet in a freshly made solution of potassium permanganate (5 grains to a quart of water). This should be done as continuously as possible for 24 to 36 hours and then 3 or 4 times a day.

The shoes and stockings of persons infected with athlete's foot should be disinfected. Stockings can be boiled. Shoes are best wiped out with a sponge wet in ether. Or they may be rinsed out at night with a 5 or 10 per cent solution of formaldehyde and allowed to dry.

Ringworm on the surface of the feet or the body may be treated with tincture of iodine unless the part is sore and irritated. Toenails infected with ringworm should be scraped with a rough piece of glass or filed to remove as much of the fungus as possible. Then they may be soaked in a solution of bichloride of mercury *or* painted with iodine. *Never apply preparations of mercury and iodine together*. Such a combination will produce a burn. X-ray treatment of infected nails gives the best prospect of cure.

"*Dhobie's itch*" is the name given to ringworm infection, supposed to be conveyed through clothing laundered by the dhobie, or Indian washerman. Red patches with a festooned edge occur in moist parts of the skin, such as the armpit and the crotch.

The nonirritating sweat-acid ointments such as Desenex ointment are excellent for this condition, whether acute or chronic. Or, for acutely irritated conditions, dressings soaked in potassium permanganate solution may be used, followed by drying and the application of talcum powder. Only when there is no irritation should tincture of iodine or Whitfield's ointment, diluted with an equal part of vaseline, be employed.

Some cases, thought to be dhobie's itch, have proved to be due to contact with the kind of ink used by the dhobie for marking garments.

Ringworm of the scalp is common among young boys in the tropics. It disappears spontaneously at puberty. It is characterized by scaly patches in which there are brittle, unhealthy hairs, broken off near the roots. The hair should be kept short or shaved, and should be shampooed once a day with warm water and mild soap. Razors, combs, scissors and towels used become infectious and should not be used by others. Treatment by X-ray is advised, when available. Sweat-acid ointments are often effective, or ammoniated mercury ointment may be applied after loose hairs have been pulled out. The infected child should wear a tight fitting muslin cap which can easily be boiled, to avoid infecting other children.

Impetigo contagiosa is an extremely contagious bacterial infection that often occurs in epidemic form among school children. It can be recognized by the honey-colored crusts adhering loosely to the skin. Treatment begins with repeated cleansing of the infected part with soap and water, removing as much of the crusts as possible. After this, a fresh solution of penicillin (500 to 1000 Oxford Units in normal saline) applied several times daily gets the best results, but this treatment should not be continued for more than a week. Ammoniated mercury ointment has long been a stand-by for such cases and continues to be useful. Ointments containing sulfa drugs are effective; but application of these drugs to the skin should be avoided whenever possible because of their frequent sensitizing effects.

Tropical ulcers (phagedena) are severe ulcers caused by various kinds of germs. They should not be confused with the "Oriental sores" of leishmaniasis. Scratches or insect bites may permit entrance of infection, usually about the ankles or on the front of the shin. The first sign of infection is often a blister. This ruptures and a large, foul-smelling sore develops.

Treatment includes provision of a nourishing diet, rich in vitamins, as well as rest and general care of the health. Whenever possible a change of climate is advised. Locally, the first problem to be met is the removal of the foul smelling, dead tissue on the surface of the sore. This may be done by surgical means. Dr. Paul Harrison, after treating large numbers of these ulcers in the humid climate of Maskat, Arabia, learned that a similar result could be obtained painlessly by applying "raw applesauce" which he made by mixing dehydrated apple powder with water.[1] After being immersed in this mixture for a few days the ulcers became clean. Then he applied a dressing, wet in cod liver oil and held tightly in place by an adhesive elastic bandage.

In small ulcers it is sometimes effective to strap the affected part with adhesive plaster, applied directly to the ulcer. After five days the plaster is pulled off and much of the dead tissue comes with it.

Wet dressings of penicillin, as directed in treatment of impetigo, are recommended for tropical ulcer. Lotions of potassium permanganate or a 5 per cent copper sulfate solution have also been used with success. Sulfa ointments may be used as a last resort.

Veld sore (desert sore) is usually caused by infection with the diphtheria bacillus. A blister forms and ruptures, leaving a raw, tender surface. In the chronic stage the ulcer is round, bluish, with thickened margins and a "punched out" appearance. After a few weeks, local paralysis of near-by muscles may be noticed. When possible, a physician will inject 4000 units of antidiphtheria serum in the vicinity of the sores. Wet dressings of penicillin solution are effective, in addition to this, and sulfanilamide powder may be used as an alternate choice.

Scabies or "itch" is common where people must live crowded together and without facilities for personal cleanliness. The disease is extremely contagious, and can be transmitted by con-

[1] Paul W. Harrison, M.D., *Doctor in Arabia* (The John Day Company).

tact with towels, bedding or clothing used by infected persons. The itching is caused by a female mite, just visible to the eye, which burrows into the skin forming a tunnel in which to lay its eggs. Itching usually begins about one hour after retiring at night and is largely confined to the front part of the body. Diagnosis is confirmed by examination of the webs between the fingers where the mite's presence is indicated by short, dirty looking marks, each ending in a blister the size of a pin head. Such burrows can be seen also on the backs of the hands, the elbows, the breast or about the groin or genitals.

In treatment the affected person should soak himself in a hot bath and then scrub the skin with soap and water, employing a stiff nail brush to lay open the burrows. After this an emulsion containing 25 to 35 per cent of benzyl benzoate is the best remedy. This is to be rubbed or painted all over the skin, excepting the face. After ten minutes the application is repeated. The medication should remain on the skin for 12 hours and then be washed off. One treatment should be sufficient.

The old-fashioned treatment of scabies with 10 per cent sulfur ointment is still used in some cases. After the scrubbing and soaking described, sulfur ointment is rubbed into the skin for a period of 20 minutes. This is done three nights in succession.

Clothing and bedclothes used by a person with scabies should be sterilized by boiling or by steam.

Lice (pediculi) are of three varieties: the head louse, the body louse, and the crab louse. *Head lice* are usually discovered because of itching of the scalp, irritation of the back of the neck or swelling of the rear neck glands. Ten per cent DDT in powder, applied to the scalp every ten days is an effective remedy. If the old-fashioned remedy of kerosene is used for application to the scalp it should be diluted with an equal part of olive oil to prevent irritation. Fire hazards should also be remembered.

Body lice live in the seams of garments. Deep, parallel scratch marks and small red points caused by bites are seen mostly on the back and shoulders. DDT powder should be applied inside garments with careful attention to the seams.

For the skin itself a bath with soap and water is usually sufficient. Unless DDT is used, all clothing worn in contact with
the skin and all bed sheets must be boiled for an hour.

Crab lice appear like black dots, partly buried at the site of
hairs in any hairy part of the body except the scalp. DDT is
very useful in treatment. Cuprex is another effective remedy
which may be used either for crab lice or head lice. All clothing in contact with the infested parts should be boiled for an
hour.

Chiggers (jiggers or chigoes) of the variety found in tropical
parts of Africa and some other countries are reddish brown
insects which resemble fleas. They attack all warm blooded
animals, but only the pregnant female burrows under the skin
where it then enlarges to the size of a pea. Pus forms, the skin
ulcerates and the chigger is finally expelled, leaving a sore
which may become seriously infected. From one chigger to
several hundred may be present at a time. The feet are most
commonly affected but other parts of the body may be involved. Prevention consists of keeping dwellings and places
where live stock and poultry are housed free from accumula-
tions of dust and dirt. After thorough sweeping these places
may be sprinkled with a solution of carbolic acid, naphthaline,
powdered tobacco, DDT, or other insecticides. Pigs and other
infested animals should not be kept in the vicinity of dwellings. Before pitching camp, sweep and spray the ground with
insecticide.

For personal protection the repellents dimethyl phthalate
or dibutyl phthalate may be applied to the feet. Or the toes
may be annointed with vaseline to which lysol or cresol has
been added in the proportion of 5 drops to the ounce. When
chiggers have penetrated the skin they should be removed as
soon as possible. Touching the chigger with a lighted cigarette or match facilitates removal. Chesterman recommends
using two blunt safety pins to enlarge the opening and remove
the skin from the chigger, rather than vice versa. A drop of
antiseptic may be applied afterward, or if infection has already
occurred the part should be soaked in a hot antiseptic solution,
such as bichloride of mercury or lysol.

Infestation by maggots, in wounds or other accessible parts may be treated by applying 5 to 10 per cent chloroform in olive oil for 30 minutes, then irrigating the part with salt solution (1 teaspoonful of salt to a cup of water). When a maggot occupies a swelling like a boil, do not try to force it out by squeezing; place a piece of fresh adhesive plaster over the opening at the apex of the swelling. Threatened with suffocation, the maggot will emerge to breathe.

Creeping eruption is caused by certain worms which burrow under the skin producing a red line which advances a little further every day. Freezing the spot with carbon dioxide snow or ethyl chloride spray or the application of an electric needle will kill the worm.

Leeches are encountered either in the water of ponds or sluggish streams or clinging to grass or leaves in jungle or grass lands. They attach themselves to the victim and suck his blood. Prolonged bleeding or infection may result. The bite is painless and may not be noticed. Repellents such as 612 and dimethyl phthalate are effective for prevention. When you are walking through forests, high boots or close fitting leggings offer some protection. An attached leech can be removed by applying salt, vinegar, or tincture of iodine to its body or holding a lighted cigarette or match near its posterior end.

[17]

DISEASES OF THE EYE

EYE INFECTIONS are transmitted by fingers, flies and infected towels or other materials used to wipe the eyes. If the eye must be rubbed, use a clean handkerchief or tissue; or, failing that, the back of the wrist. Never touch the eyes with unwashed fingers. Adequate screening and use of insecticides will provide reasonably effective protection against flies. Small children can be protected when outside by attaching veils to their hat brims.

Refrain from rubbing the eye when a foreign body in it causes discomfort. After washing the hands grasp the upper eye lashes and pull the lid down over the lower one. If this is unsuccessful, wash the eye out with boric acid lotion or clean water. In case irritation continues after this, the eyeball itself and the lining (conjunctiva) of both lids must be inspected, by everting (turning inside out) first the upper lid, then the lower lid. The upper lid can be readily everted with the aid of a lead pencil. To do this, grasp the lashes between the thumb and index finger of the left hand. Direct the patient to look downward as the lid is pulled down and away from the eye. Now, with the right hand, place the lead of the pencil horizontally in line with the fold of the upper lid. As the lead is pushed downward, pull the lashes and margin of the eyelid upward. The lid is thus everted. If possible, use a magnifying glass when looking for a foreign body. If a body is seen either on the upper lid, lower lid, or the front of the eyeball, remove it with a cotton applicator moistened with water.

When nothing avails for removing a foreign body and no physician can be called, put a drop of mineral oil or other bland oil into the eye, and bandage lightly, trusting that nature will in time remove the irritant. When a chemical substance such as battery fluid or alkaline cleansing powder gets into the eye it should be washed out immediately with cupful after cupful of milk or water. Then drop bland oil into the eye and apply cold compresses.

In cases of injury to the eyeball, the victim should see a doctor as soon as possible. In the meantime put a small amount of antibiotic ointment, such as terramycin, aureomycin, or bacitracin, into the eye and bandage firmly. If no medical aid is available repeat the instillation every three hours.

Styes are abscesses resulting from infection of small glands at the edges of the eyelids. Becoming red, swollen, and painful, they finally come to a head and discharge pus. Poor health or eyestrain may predispose to such a condition. When a series of styes occurs, one should try to find the underlying cause. "Ripening" of the abscess may be hastened by the use of compresses kept hot for thirty minutes, four times a day. A physician may incise the swelling, but in the absence of medical aid it is better to wait for the abscess to break spontaneously. Do not squeeze a stye at any time.

Chronic inflammation of the edges of the eyelids (blepharitis). In one form this consists of simple scaliness, a condition resembling dandruff in the scalp. In another form, "granular lids," yellow crusts glue the lashes together. Local treatment of granular lids begins with removal of the crusts after softening with white Vaseline or mineral oil. The edges of the lids should then be treated with an antibiotic ophthalmic ointment, rubbed on the lid margins with an applicator.

Trachoma is a disease characterized by granular inflammation of the lining of the eyelids. It is extremely contagious, and should be suspected whenever lids appear chronically red and swollen and eyes watery and unhealthy looking. In order to diagnose trachoma, the lids must be everted and their lining examined. Hands must be washed immediately after this procedure.

In early stages of trachoma the mucous membrane lining the lids, instead of being normally smooth and glistening, is thick and velvety with sometimes a granular or pebbled appearance. Later, translucent follicles like small grains of cooked sago or tapioca may stand out from the general surface. These irritate the eye. Pus may form, due to secondary infection. In chronic cases scar tissue on the lining of the lids contracts, causing the eyelashes to scrape the eyeball. This often leads to blindness. An operation on the lids is indicated.

Treatment of trachoma is by the use of antibiotics and sulfonamides (sulfa drugs). A physician may give large doses of sulfonamides internally and antibiotics, usually in ointment form, locally. The lay worker should confine himself to local treatment, applying an antibiotic ophthalmic ointment every four hours.

Conjunctivitis is inflammation of the conjunctiva, the delicate membrane covering the surface of the eyeball as well as lining the lids. It is indicated by redness and a discharge which often contains pus. This is contagious if the ordinary rules of cleanliness are not observed.

Severe cases of conjunctivitis are very common in the tropics. Greatly swollen, painful eyes, filled with pus are an everyday sight. Many cases are due to infection by flies, especially in countries where there is a season for "eye flies." In some instances the inflammation may be due to germs of gonorrhea, conveyed either by fingers contaminated with discharge from an infected person, or in ophthalmia of the new born, from contact of the infant's eyes with an infected birth canal.

In severe infections the eyelids often become glued together with pus. Unless the examiner is very careful when separating the lids he may be hit in the eye by a stream of the discharge. In other cases the conjunctiva of the lids becomes so swollen and inflamed that the eyelids become everted and appear like fiery, red plums lying on the face at the site of the eyes.

A patient with severe conjunctivitis is really ill. He should stay in bed, be seen by a doctor as soon as possible and receive careful nursing.

Preparation for nursing care of eye infections should receive adequate thought. The attendant must avoid infecting his own eyes, the eyes of others with whom he may have contact and the patient's healthy eye, in case only one eye is affected. It will help him to have things conveniently arranged. Not far from the patient's bed or the place of treatment should be facilities for washing the hands: soap and water, a nail brush and a supply of paper towels or other small towels which can easily be boiled after use. If rubber gloves are not available, there should also be a basin containing rubbing alcohol or a solution of bichloride of mercury in which to soak the hands after thorough scrubbing.

It will be convenient to have all bottles and other objects used in the treatments arranged on a tray to be kept near at hand and covered with a clean towel when not in use. Patented all-glass drop-bottles which prevent the necessity for using medicine droppers are convenient for containing lotions and eye drops. If droppers are to be used they should be boiled before and after use and kept in a sterile container. Glass jars with covers, such as those in which mayonnaise is purchased, make convenient receptacles. They can be placed in a kettle of cold water, boiled for ten minutes and then allowed to dry by evaporation. Other jars of this sort can be used for small balls or pledgets of absorbent cotton or cotton applicators. A pair of long forceps (or a fork), to be used for removing these articles from the jars, should be sterilized and then kept in a tall jar with its blades (or prongs) immersed in alcohol. If a "kidney basin" is obtainable it should also be kept on the tray. The patient can hold it against his cheek to catch the overflow when an eye is irrigated. This basin should be boiled after use for infective cases. For receiving soiled cotton and swabs a waste basket lined with a paper bag should be kept near the bed. Contents are to be burned with the bag, avoiding contact of infective material with the fingers.

Dangerous infections of the eye often begin very suddenly and without warning. Travelers expecting to live beyond the range of prompt medical assistance need to be prepared for emergencies of this kind. Intelligent, faithful care by a lay attendant while waiting for a doctor to arrive can do much to save eyes whose eyesight might otherwise be lost.

Pus forming in an eye should be washed out. Adult patients can, if necessary, be taught to help themselves in this respect if a bowl of eye lotion and a supply of small balls of absorbent cotton, together with a receptacle for soiled cotton and facilities for washing and disinfecting the hands are placed within their reach. Warm boric acid lotion, bichloride of mercury lotion (1:5000), or even plain, boiled water may be used for this purpose. A minimum of six such cleansings should be given in a day. A fresh piece of cotton should be used for wiping each infected eye. A bandage should never be applied to an eye in which there is pus.

Whenever possible patients with severe eye infections should be isolated. In very severe infections if only one eye is infected great care must be taken to protect the other eye. One device for protecting the uninfected eye is the "Buller's shield," commonly used in ophthalmia of the newborn. The latter consists of a watch glass fitted in a square piece of adhesive plaster which is carefully applied to the brow, temple, lower margin of the orbit and nose of the healthy eye. This should be secured with additional strips to prevent the entrance of discharge. The inner margin is sealed with collodion, since contamination is most likely to occur at this point; and inefficient application increases, rather than diminishes, the danger.

If a Buller's shield is unavailable it may be possible to apply a gauze dressing, the edges of which are made tight by fastening along them strips of gauze painted with flexible collodion. At any rate, the patient should be instructed to sleep on the infected side to avoid the downward flow of secretion into the uninfected eye.

To reduce swelling, ice-cold compresses may be applied for a half hour, four times a day; or the doctor may prescribe hot applications under certain circumstances. In addition, antibiotic ophthalmic ointment should be applied every three hours.

Corneal ulcers are ulcers in the transparent tissue, the cornea, which lies over the colored part of the eye. In the presence of an ulcer it may be very difficult to inspect the eye because of painful spasm on attempt to open the eye. The doctor usually applies a local anesthetic inside the eye. The lay worker, in case no doctor is available, may use a ½ per cent solution of pontocaine for this purpose. The patient is told to "look up" and the lower lid is pulled down so that the everted lid forms a shelf, and one drop of this solution is instilled into the eye. Three drops in succession are to be used in this way at intervals of ½ minute, the patient keeping his eyes closed between instillations.

After the pontocaine solution has produced anesthesia it should be possible to inspect the cornea. An ulcer may be recognized as a white or yellowish white opaque spot which is less shiny than the rest of the cornea. It is very urgent to secure medical help if an ulcer is present. If this is impossible apply antibiotic ophthalmic ointment in the eye every three hours. The eye should be kept bandaged between the instillations of the ointment.

MALARIA AND BLACKWATER FEVER

·····································

MALARIA

MALARIA is a disease characterized by periodic attacks of fever, accompanied by anemia and enlargement of the spleen. It is at present the greatest disease problem and the chief cause of death throughout the world. It is found practically everywhere, except in the frigid zone, but its frequency and virulence increase as the equator is approached.

CAUSE

MALARIA is due to infection with malaria parasites transmitted by the bite of female anopheles mosquitoes. In general this mosquito differs from other varieties in that it has spotted wings and a straight body which forms an angle of 45° with the surface on which it rests. Of 160 known species of anophelines at least 30 have been found to transmit malaria. For the complete life cycle of the parasite of human malaria both a human being and an anopheles mosquito are necessary. Infection can, however, be transferred from one human being to another by transfusion of blood or the use of a hypodermic needle contaminated with the blood of an infected person.

The degree of malaria in a community can be estimated by two methods:

1. The *parasitic index:* Persons trained in microscopic diagnosis of malaria can form an estimate of the extent to which a community is infected by examining the blood of a large number of the inhabitants. Many adults who have no

138

symptoms may be found to harbor the disease. The percentage figure showing the proportion of specimens containing parasites, in relation to the total number examined, is the parasitic index.

2. The *splenic index* can be ascertained by lay workers. It is obtained by discovering the percentage of native children, between the ages of two and ten years, who have enlarged spleens. With the child standing and taking a deep breath as he faces the examiner the latter inserts his hand beneath the lowest rib on the left side of the abdomen. Normally no solid object is felt in this location. An enlarged spleen on the other hand, gives a feeling of resistance. The mass extends a few inches below the rib, or even in severe cases, seems almost to fill the abdomen.

In choosing a place to reside in the tropics the use of the splenic index may be of great practical importance. If 50 per cent of children examined in the locality have large spleens the place may be considered extremely malarious and dangerous. A rate of 25 to 50 per cent shows the disease to be very prevalent. With 10 to 25 per cent of large spleens the disease is moderately prevalent. A locality with less than 10 per cent is considered comparatively healthful.

PREVENTION

THIS MAY be considered under three headings:
1. The extermination of mosquitoes.
2. The prevention of infection of people by mosquitoes.
3. The prevention of infection of mosquitoes by people.

1. *Extermination of mosquitoes:*

(a) *Elimination of Breeding Places.* Information as to the most important measures to be used in any area can be obtained from the local health officers. What is useful in one location may be actually harmful in another place where a different kind of anopheles mosquito transmits malaria. Sometimes the indicated measure is to cut down brush and let in sunlight, while in other places it is just the opposite, i.e. to provide shade which the local important malarial mosquito cannot endure. Drainage is always useful, but it is usually expensive.

Filling in depressions which collect water is always useful but is more expensive. Cleaning vegetation away from the edges of standing or running water is usually advantageous because it removes the shelter of vegetation from anopheles larvae and makes them accessible to their natural enemies.

(*b*) *Destruction of Mosquito Larvae.* Formerly this was accomplished through the application of either oil or Paris green to the surface of water where mosquitoes breed. Now it will usually be possible to employ DDT in diesel oil. It is said that the use of two quarts of 5 per cent diesel oil solution of DDT is as effective in killing larvae as 20 to 40 gallons of oil without DDT. On a large scale, DDT is sometimes dispersed by airplane.

Another means of destroying mosquito larvae is by the introduction of small fish which are the natural enemies of larvae. Thus gambusia are useful in the rice fields of Egypt. Minnows are also found in rice fields and are said to live through the winter in ditches and canals. Gold fish destroy larvae in garden ponds.

(*c*) *Destruction of Adult Mosquitoes.* Insecticide sprays, such as those containing pyrethrum have long been so used. DDT has an outstanding contribution as an insecticide because of its *long-lasting residual effects.* Although it acts more slowly than pyrethrum its anti-malaria value against adult mosquitoes is enormous in that it kills them before their infection can reach the infective stage. An amazing reduction in the incidence of malaria in Panama has been achieved by the spraying of native huts inside and out with DDT three or four times a year. In this case 400 mg. of DDT was employed per square foot of space. The mosquitoes apparently rest on the walls of the huts after flight and after biting and absorb the DDT through their feet.

In the household DDT can be used in emulsion form to spray walls, screens of doors and windows and to impregnate netting used for bed curtains. Mosquito bombs containing DDT will be useful on occasion.

2. *Prevention of infection of people* by mosquitoes. This is accomplished by:

(a) Screening of houses or *at least* of sleeping rooms.

(b) Use of bed nets.

(c) Use of repellents such as the 6–2–2 mixture, as explained in chapter 8.

(d) Protective clothing for those who must be outside screened houses at night. Mosquito boots, long trousers and sleeves, gloves and headnets are recommended.

3. *Prevention of infection of mosquitoes* by people is achieved chiefly by having all infected persons sleep under nets. "Don't infect the mosquito and the mosquito can't infect you."

What Is Suppressive Treatment?

Suppressive treatment, although sometimes called "prophylaxis" is not a true preventive. No drug known at present is able to kill the malaria organism as soon as it is injected by a mosquito. But malaria can be *suppressed* so that no symptoms occur. During World War II atabrine was the drug employed to keep armed forces free of symptoms. Formerly quinine had been used. Newer drugs are now replacing atabrine, which is a dye and imparts a yellow color to the skin.

Should those who plan to live for years in a malarious locality begin on arrival, or before arrival, to take medicine for suppressive treatment?

Doctors disagree on this subject. Residents who have the advantage of medical supervision should defer to their doctors' judgment in this matter. For any lay persons who must take the responsibility for preventing illness in a malarious locality the following plans for suppressive treatment are given. Treatment may be started two weeks before exposure is anticipated and should be continued for at least a month after leaving the district.

SUPPRESSIVE TREATMENT WITH ARALEN (CHLOROQUINE)

(See Appendix C)

Tablets contain 0.25 gram (base 0.15 gram)

ADULTS

2 tablets (0.5 gram) once a week continuously, on the same day of the week, if in a highly malarious area.

CHILDREN (*according to age*)

0–1 year	¼ tablet	(0.062 gram [1 grain])
1–3 years	½ "	(0.125 gram [2 grains])
3–6 years	¾ "	(0.18 gram [3 grains])
6–10 years	1 "	(0.25 gram [4 grains])
10–14 years	1½ "	(0.375 gram [5 grains])

The dose indicated in the above table is to be given once a week; i.e., for an infant ¼ tablet once a week; for a child of 8 years, 1 tablet weekly.

SUPPRESSIVE TREATMENT WITH PALUDRINE OR GUANATOL

(See Appendix C)

ADULTS

1 tablet containing 0.1 gram (1½ grain) twice a week, 3–4 days apart—continuously or during the malarial season. If this does not prove effective, take one tablet on alternate days or even daily.

CHILDREN

Use tablets containing only 25 or 50 milligrams.

0–1 year	½ of a 25 mgm. tablet *twice* a week
1–3 years	1	25 mgm. tablet *twice* a week
3–6 years	1½	25 mgm. tablet *twice* a week
6–9 years	1	50 mgm. tablet *twice* a week
9–12 years	1½	50 mgm. tablet *twice* a week
Over 12 years	1	100 mgm. (0.1 gram) tablet *twice* a week

SUPPRESSIVE TREATMENT WITH ATABRINE (QUINACRINE)

ADULTS

0.1 gram (1½ grains) daily

CHILDREN (*according to age*)

0–2 years	0.025 gram (⅓ grain) every second day
3–8 years	0.025 gram (⅓ grain) daily
8–15 years	0.05 gram (1 grain) daily
15 years or over, adult dose	

SUPPRESSIVE TREATMENT WITH QUININE

ADULTS

0.32 gram (5 grains) daily

CHILDREN (*according to age*)

Less than 1 year	0.017 gram	(¼ grain) daily
1 year	0.032 gram	(½ grain) daily
2 years	0.065 gram	(1 grain) daily
3–4 years	0.125 gram	(2 grains) daily
5–7 years	0.2 gram	(3 grains) daily
8–10 years	0.25 gram	(4 grains) daily

10 years or over, adult dose

Instead of quinine for suppressive treatment in children it is the custom in some places to administer a daily dose of euquinine (quinine ethyl carbonate), a powder containing 59 per cent of quinine alkaloid. This is preferred by some because of its less bitter taste. It is often administered, mixed with jam or honey. The dose is the same as that of quinine, or a little larger.

The Role of Health Education in Preventing Malaria

Cooperation of the general population is greatly to be desired in the project of freeing any community from malaria. The extreme poverty of many of the inhabitants of countries where malaria is common interferes to a discouraging degree however with results of health education. It should be the aim to have every person sleep under a bed net; but often this is impossible and all that can be hoped for is to produce intelligent cooperation with government agencies whose business is the eradication or oiling of standing water, spraying of houses and vehicles and other public health measures. The cinema is a useful means of disseminating information to both adults and children.[1]

---

[1] Walt Disney's film on malaria, called *Winged Scourge* can be obtained from the Institute of Inter-American Affairs, Washington, D.C.

TYPES OF MALARIA

MALARIA is either "benign" or "malignant."

Benign types are (1) benign tertian malaria, a common form due to the Plasmodium vivax, whose symptoms often, but not always, occur every third day (i.e. at intervals of forty-eight hours); (2) quartan malaria, due to the Plasmodium malariae, whose symptoms occur every fourth day and (3) malaria due to the Plasmodium ovale, a less common type whose symptoms occur every forty-eight hours.

The *malignant* form of malaria, due to the Plasmodium falciparum, is called "malignant tertian," "subtertian" or "aestivo autumnal" malaria. It has a cycle of about forty-eight hours but is often irregular.

It is not always possible to distinguish types of malaria by the intervals at which symptoms occur. The patient may have been infected more than once with the same or different kinds of parasite. Fever is called "remittent" when paroxysms overlap and fever occurs every day, or "intermittent" when free intervals occur.

Benign tertian malaria, although not usually dangerous to life is very difficult to cure and usually relapses. Malignant malaria, although more dangerous to life if untreated, can usually be cured by the treatments to be outlined.

Persons accustomed to relapses of malaria should, for years, always take anti-malaria medicine with them when traveling. They can recognize the beginning of symptoms and take the medicine at once.

SYMPTOMS

SYMPTOMS of malaria are often misleading. The first attack of the benign type is often far from typical. Fever may be continuous. A relapse may simulate anything from acute appendicitis to lobar pneumonia. Persons accustomed to relapses should never be without anti-malaria medicine. They should take this, when unable to secure medical advice, no matter what their symptoms are. And no matter what other disease is present malaria is always likely to be a complicating factor.

Symptoms of a Typical Attack of Benign Tertian Malaria

In this, the most common and mildest type, there are in typical cases three stages of symptoms:

1. *Cold stage* (duration ½ to 2 hours): This stage may be preceded by a headache, a tired feeling, lack of appetite and muscular pains. In other cases a violent chill begins abruptly. The teeth chatter, the body shakes the bed, the skin is dusky and cold, goose flesh appears and the lips are blue and the features pinched. In spite of coldness of the surface the temperature may rise to 104°–105° in this stage. Headache and vomiting are common.

2. *Hot stage* (duration 3 to 5 hours): The sensation of coldness gradually gives way to one of warmth, followed by intense heat. Fever may reach 106°. The pulse is full and fast. Fever blisters sometimes occur on the lips. The patient suffers from restlessness, headache, muscular pains and thirst. There may be slight delirium.

3. *Sweating stage* (duration 1 to 2 hours): Now the temperature falls. Sweating is profuse. Pains disappear and thirst abates. The patient falls into a refreshing sleep. After he awakes he may go about his work as usual, feeling perhaps, a little languid.

Enlargement of the spleen: The spleen is almost always enlarged during the chill. Tenderness over the region of the spleen is usually present during the stage of fever. After many attacks the spleen remains large. This condition is called "ague cake."

Symptoms in small children are often atypical. Convulsions may take the place of a chill and sweating may be absent. There may be diarrhea and vomiting.

Symptoms of Malignant Malaria

These are more severe than those of other types. Fever may last for more than twenty-four hours without a break. It may begin in the late afternoon and continue throughout the following day.

The chill is less marked than in the other types. Severe digestive disturbances sometimes occur and anemia and emaciation may be extreme.

Pernicious Malaria

This term refers to special and very dangerous manifestations of malaria which are usually, but not always, due to infection with the malignant parasite. Various types of symptoms occur, according to the part of the body in which the parasites lodge.

1. *The gastro-intestinal form* is sometimes mistaken for cholera, food-poisoning, gall-bladder disease, appendicitis or ruptured ulcer of the stomach. There may be pain, diarrhea and vomiting. Blood is sometimes vomited or passed from the rectum. The disease may resemble bacillary dysentery.

2. *The cerebral form,* in which parasites lodge in the brain, causes severe headache, drowsiness and unconsciousness from which the patient cannot be aroused. There may be vomiting. Paralysis may also occur.

3. *The algid type* is one in which infection is so overwhelming that the patient dies after six or eight hours without fever having occurred. The temperature may even be subnormal. The surface of the body is cold and clammy, the eyes are sunken and collapse is profound.

4. Other pernicious types may simulate pneumonia, kidney disease or almost any kind of serious illness.

Latent Malaria

This term describes a condition in which parasites live in the body for a long time without producing symptoms. Eventually symptoms may be precipitated by fatigue, cold and wet, injury, operation or childbirth. Chills and fever from this cause, occurring after operation or childbirth, are sometimes mistaken for blood poisoning. A person who has, for a long time, been free of symptoms of malaria while living in the tropics is likely to have an attack of fever after reaching a cooler climate.

Very severe anemia may result from destruction of red blood cells by malaria parasites. In some cases the patient has not been known to be suffering from malaria. This anemia calls for treatment with iron. Extremely anemic patients should move away from the malarial district. With appropriate treatment they may recover.

TREATMENT OF MALARIA

1. *Put the patient to bed* as soon as he feels chilly, preferably before actual shivering begins. Supply hot water bottles and hot drinks and cover him warmly.

2. *Secure a diagnosis:* If it is at all possible to secure medical help, wait for the doctor to take a specimen of blood for examination before giving any anti-malaria drug. In some places where medical service is not quickly available lay persons can be taught to make a "spread" from a drop of blood taken from the finger or the lobe of the ear. Two glass slides should be prepared in this way and put aside until their examination is possible. If anti-malaria medicine has been given *before* the spreads are made, laboratory tests will probably be useless since all the malaria parasites will have disappeared from the blood.

3. *If no medical help for diagnosis and treatment can be secured and the patient is thought to have malaria begin treatment with an anti-malaria drug as soon as possible.* The other anti-malaria drugs are to be preferred to quinine for the pregnant and those who for some reason cannot take quinine.

TREATMENT OF ACUTE ATTACKS OF MALARIA WITH ARALEN

(See Appendix C)

ADULTS
Single dose is 2 tablets, each containing 0.25 gram (base 0.15).
Course: 4 tablets taken at once
        2 tablets 6 hours later
        2 tablets daily for 2 days
        Total: 10 tablets taken within 3 days (2.5 grams)
CHILDREN
0–1 year: Initial dose, 1 tablet (0.25 gram) followed by 1 tablet (0.25 gram) 6 hours later. Total, 0.50 gram.
2–5 years: Initial dose, 2 tablets (0.50 gram) followed by 1 tablet (0.25 gram) 8 hours later. Total, 0.75 gram.

6–10 years: Initial dose, 2 tablets (0.50 gram) plus two doses of 1 tablet with 8-hour interval. Total, 1.0 gram.

11–15 years: Initial dose, 3 tablets (0.75 gram) followed by 1 tablet (0.25 gram) 8 hours later and 1 tablet (0.25 gram) 24 hours later. Total, 1.25 gram.

TREATMENT OF ACUTE ATTACKS OF MALARIA WITH PALUDRINE OR GUANATOL
(See Appendix C)

ADULTS

If the infection is known to be due to *malignant (Falciparum) parasites,* a single dose of 3 tablets (0.1 gram each) will abort an attack. For radical cure: 1 tablet (0.1 gram) three times a day for 10 days, or twice a day for 14 days. In *benign tertian malaria (Vivax)* a single dose of 3 tablets will bring the temperature to normal, and relapses may be prevented by taking 1 tablet (0.1 gram) twice a week, 3 or 4 days apart.

The *best course when the type of infection is unknown,* is to take 1 tablet 3 times a day for 10 days, then 1 tablet twice a week for 3 months.

CHILDREN (*based on* apparent *age*)

0–1 year	½	of a 25 mgm. (0.025 gram) tablet twice a day
1–3 years	1	25 mgm. tablet twice a day
3–6 years	1	25 mgm. tablet 3 times a day
6–9 years	1	50 mgm. tablet twice a day
9–12 years	1	50 mgm. tablet 3 times a day
12–15 years	1	100 mgm. tablet twice a day
Over 15 years	1	100 mgm. tablet 3 times a day

If necessary the larger tablets may be cut in sections of a quarter or a half to secure the approximate dose indicated. Using these doses, appropriate for the age, the course should be given as in the case of adults.

TREATMENT OF MALARIA WITH ATABRINE

ADULTS

2 tablets (each 0.1 gram, or 1½ grains) thrice daily, *after meals* for 2 days.

After this, 1 tablet thrice daily, *after meals,* for 5 days. When the drug causes digestive disturbance each dose may be accompanied by ¼ teaspoonful of bicarbonate of soda (baking soda). Atabrine should never be given on an empty stomach.

CHILDREN

For young children tablets should be crushed and combined with syrup or honey.

Up to 1 year ¼ tablet (0.025 gram or ⅜ grain) twice daily for 5 days

1–4 years ½ tablet (0.05 gram or ¾ grain) twice daily for 5 days

4–8 years 1 tablet (0.1 gram or 1½ grain) twice daily for 5 days

8–12 years 1 tablet (0.1 gram or 1½ grain) thrice daily for 5 days

12 years or over, adult dose

TREATMENT OF MALARIA WITH QUININE

ADULTS

Of quinine sulphate [1] or the soluble bihydrochloride 10 grains, in either uncoated tablets, capsules or solution, thrice daily for 3 days. Then 10 grains twice daily for a week. After this, 10 grains once daily for 3 weeks.

CHILDREN

Under 1 year approximately, $\frac{1}{10}$ the adult dose

1–2 years ⅛ the adult dose

2–6 years ¼ the adult dose

6–12 years ½ the adult dose

12 years or over, adult dose

The Intravenous Injection of Quinine. For serious illness with malaria, and especially in case of pernicious types of the disease, a physician may inject quinine bihydrochloride intravenously.

The Intramuscular Injection of Quinine. The possibility of injecting quinine intramuscularly should be mentioned. This method is far inferior to use of the intravenous route. Occasionally it gives rise to considerable soreness or even abscess formation at the site of injection. Nevertheless, in the hands of an attendant who is unable to give intravenous injections it may be the means of saving lives. When a patient is very ill with malaria and cannot take quinine by mouth or receive it

[1] One drop of concentrated hydrochloric acid will cause 5 grains of quinine sulphate to dissolve in a teaspoonful of water.

by intravenous injection, 10 grains of quinine bihydrochloride, in the form of tablets especially prepared for injection, may be dissolved in 5 cc. of boiled water and injected into the buttock. The upper, outer quadrant of the buttock is the preferred location. The syringe should be boiled before use and the skin painted with an antiseptic. After the injection the tissues should be massaged gently to promote absorption. Injections may be made into the two buttocks alternately, 1 to 3 times a day according to the urgency of the patient's condition. As soon as medicines can be taken by mouth injections should be discontinued.

Quinine, Given by Enema. When no other way of administering quinine is possible it may be injected into the rectum. A lay person could use the following directions:

After a cleansing enema an adult may be given 2 grams (30 grains) of quinine in solution (preferably the bihydrochloride) diluted with 3–10 ounces of liquid starch, prepared as follows:

Mix one teaspoonful of laundry starch with a little cold water. Stir until smooth. Then add hot water until mucilage is formed. The mixture should be introduced as high into the rectum as possible, using a tube or catheter instead of a nozzle. The patient should be kept quiet with the hips elevated on a pillow to prevent expulsion of the liquid.

Quinine by enema is useful in treating children suffering from convulsions due to malaria. A dose of 0.3 gram (5 grains) in an ounce of liquid starch may be given to a child of one year. The buttocks should be pressed together afterward to prevent expulsion of the medication. Injections of the same strength may if necessary be repeated at hourly intervals until convulsions cease.

Undesirable Effects of Quinine Medication. Large doses of quinine often cause "ringing" in the ears and blurring of vision. These are not of serious import. Indigestion, vomiting or a skin eruption may occur in patients sensitive to the drug. In the pregnant quinine has been thought to bring on miscarriage. But malaria *must* be treated in the pregnant and, with care, quinine may safely be given when other drugs are not available. The following plan of *desensitizing* a patient who for some reason finds it difficult to take quinine has been found useful in India.

Desensitizing doses of quinine: Begin with $\frac{1}{10}$ grain of quinine, combined with $\frac{1}{3}$ teaspoonful of baking soda. Half an hour later give $\frac{2}{10}$ grain, likewise combined with soda. Continue giving quinine and soda every half hour, doubling the amount of quinine each time until the normal dose is tolerated.

4. *General treatment of malaria:* Good nursing is very important throughout serious attacks of malaria. There should be rest in bed and constant supervision. Patients with a high temperature sometimes become maniacal and attempt suicide.

Besides the use of anti-malarial drugs other measures should be taken to *lower the temperature.* Cool sponging should be started when the fever reaches 103°. If it mounts still higher the patient should be wrapped in a sheet wrung out of tepid water or be lifted into a tub of tepid water which is afterward cooled.

For symptomatic treatment of nausea $\frac{1}{2}$ teaspoonful of baking soda may be given with a little water and repeated at intervals. *Constipation* should be relieved by a laxative. The diet should be liquid while there is fever. At other times a nourishing convalescent diet is in order. After an attack anemia should be treated with iron in medicinal form.

BLACKWATER FEVER

BLACKWATER FEVER is a complication of malignant malaria with an average mortality of 25 to 30 per cent. The disease gets its name from the fact that the urine assumes a black or dark color due to the presence of hemoglobin, the coloring matter of blood. Blackwater fever appears only in areas where malignant malaria is common and in people who have been infected for several months. Inadequate treatment of malaria seems to be a predisposing factor. On the other hand the disease seems not to occur in those who have had serious attacks of malaria accompanied by high fever. Anyone who has lived in an infected area may contract the disease; but males have proved to be more susceptible than females.

PREVENTION

IN PLACES where blackwater fever occurs care should be taken to avoid overexertion and exposure to chilling. Alcoholic drinks should not be used. Symptoms of malaria should not be overlooked or neglected, even though they are slight. The disease should be promptly and adequately treated. Attacks are often brought on by a large dose of quinine taken for a relapse of malaria after a period when treatment has been neglected.

The Pre-Blackwater State

For the benefit of those who live where blackwater fever is known to occur the following symptoms may give warning of the possible approach of the disease. The complexion becomes sallow and the whites of the eyes have a yellow tinge. The tongue is heavily coated and constipation is the rule. The urine looks darker than usual. Both the spleen and liver are enlarged and can be felt in the abdomen below the lowest rib on the left and right side respectively. There is usually headache and slight irregular fever.

The onset of actual blackwater fever is usually evidenced by a sudden rise in temperature to 103° or even higher. The fever may become irregular after this. Backache occurs, together with other aches and pains. There is an urgent desire to void and the urine becomes almost black in color. The skin is jaundiced. In severe cases there may be vomiting, discomfort in the region of the stomach and severe pain over the liver. The fever may rise to 104° or higher, the urine may become scanty and finally be suppressed altogether. Complete suppression of urine is a very unfavorable sign in regard to the prospect of recovery.

TREATMENT OF THE PRE-BLACKWATER STATE

1. As soon as the temperature rises the patient should be put to bed. It is a mistake to go about as usual, and especially dangerous to travel. Secure a physician at the earliest possible moment.

2. The skin should be kept warm and protected from draughts.

3. As much fluid as possible should be drunk in order to increase the amount of urine. Drinks should be taken warm and in small quantities. From this point until well into the convalescent period, in case blackwater fever actually develops, food should consist only of liquids, including fruit juices, broths, and milk. Acid fruit cordials should not be given.

4. Every 4 hours give a teaspoonful of baking soda dissolved in water. This need not be taken all at once but may be supplied gradually, combined with fluids taken.

TREATMENT OF BLACKWATER FEVER

1. Careful nursing is exceedingly important. The patient becomes very weak before he is able to assimilate food and even the act of sitting up in bed may precipitate heart failure.

2. It is very urgent to provide the services of a physician. In case no medical advice can be secured continue the fluid diet and the doses of baking soda. If the usual liquid foods cannot be retained try barley water and albumin water.[2] When the stomach cannot retain any fluids inject a glass full of warm salt solution into the rectum, using a teaspoonful of table salt to a glass of boiled water. Raise the hips on a pillow to enable the enema to be retained. Repeat the injection every half hour or hour.

3. If nausea occurs it may sometimes be lessened by holding cracked ice in the mouth. Vomiting may be lessened by the application of a mustard plaster or cloths wrung out of very hot water to the pit of the stomach.

A physician should decide about the resumption of suppressive treatment after an attack of blackwater fever. Other antimalaria drugs are probably safer for this purpose than quinine.

---

[2] Albumin water can be made by adding ½ cup of cold water to the white of an egg, with a teaspoon of sugar and the same amount of lemon juice, and shaking all together in a tightly closed glass fruit jar.

SOME TROPICAL FEVERS
OTHER THAN MALARIA

▬▬▬▬▬▬▬▬▬▬▬▬▬▬▬▬▬▬▬▬▬▬▬▬▬▬▬▬▬▬▬▬▬▬▬▬▬▬

Typhoid Fever

Typhoid fever (enteric fever), a disease associated with ulceration of the intestine and characterized by fever which lasts about four weeks, is found throughout the world. This disease and the similar but milder *paratyphoid fevers* are responsible for many cases of prolonged, undiagnosed cases of fever in children and adults.

The *cause* is the *typhoid bacillus* from the discharges of patients or healthy "carriers" of the disease. This contaminates food or drink.

Symptoms begin with a period of illness with headache, backache and discomfort in the abdomen. After this temperature begins to rise, then fall slightly and rise again higher than before. After about a week, the fever reaches its highest point and at the end of the third week begins to fall. After apparent recovery the patient may have a relapse, generally milder than the original attack.

Characteristic of the disease is the pulse rate which is usually 20 to 40 beats slower than would be expected with the associated degree of temperature. The face is flushed and has a dull, stuporous appearance. Delirium, if present, is of the low, muttering variety. The mouth is dry and the tongue coated in the middle, with a clean tip and edges. Diarrhea is often present but constipation may take its place; or diarrhea and constipation may occur alternately. There may be nausea and vomiting and the abdomen may be either bloated or sunken. Scattered rose-colored spots often appear on the chest and abdomen, coming out in crops, seven to ten days after the onset. These are single, slightly elevated to the touch and lose their color on pressure.

Dreaded *complications* of typhoid fever are (1) perforation of an intestinal ulcer with resulting peritonitis and (2) hemorrhage into the intestine with appearance of black or bright red blood in the stools.

Vaccination is the most effective method of *prevention*. Destruction of flies, use of safe food and drink, with handwashing before touching food and before eating are also essential modes of prevention.

Treatment. The patient should, if possible, be placed in a modern hospital. No cathartic should be used, but when necessary an enema of a pint of warm water containing a teaspoonful of salt may be given as an enema. Recently Chloromycetin has given promise of exerting a specific effect.

At least 7 or 8 pints of fluid should be drunk daily. Adequate nutrition is very important. Milk is the most valuable single article of food. Diluted fruit juices should be given unless they cause distress. Soft foods, as outlined in chapter 10, are usually well borne. Anything hard, such as toast, should be avoided. If hemorrhage takes place, food and drink should be stopped for twenty-four hours and then resumed gradually. Convalescence is lengthy and relapses are frequent.

Dengue

Dengue (dandy fever, breakbone fever, seven-day fever) occurs in rapidly spreading epidemics and is due to a virus, conveyed by the bites of mosquitoes, chiefly of the Aedes aegypti variety. Beginning with a chill followed by a rise of temperature which may reach 106°, it produces a deep flushing of the face and a rash which may be seen for an hour or more. The head and eyeballs ache, and a part or the whole of the body is racked by pain resembling rheumatism. Prostration is great and the pulse rate may be 120 or more. After a day or two. the temperature becomes normal, but on the fourth or seventh day fever and pains return, accompanied by a rash which in some ways resembles the rashes of both measles and scarlet fever. Rheumatic pains persist, sometimes for months, and relapses are common. A change of climate may be advisable, although the disease is never fatal. Prevention is through mosquito control.

In treatment, bed rest may be needed for as long as ten days. Chilling should be avoided, and a light diet is indicated. Aspirin helps in relieving the pain as does local application of oil of wintergreen to the joints. Ice water or lemonade should be given frequently during fever, and enemas are to be preferred to purgatives to relieve constipation.

Sandfly Fever (Pappataci Fever, Phlebotomus Fever)

Sandfly fever may occur wherever the sandfly is found. It is known as a fever which lasts three days and is never fatal.

Symptoms begin about four to seven days after the bite of an infected sandfly. A chill is followed by fever. The face is flushed, the front of the head aches and there is pain and stiffness in the back of the neck. Pain occurs also at the back of the eyes, which are bloodshot. The legs and back ache, the tongue is furred and the patient is drowsy but cannot sleep. In from twenty-four to thirty-six hours the temperature reaches 103° or 104°. It persists for one more day and then begins to fall. At this time nosebleed, vomiting, sweating and diarrhea may occur. At the end of the third day the temperature is usually normal; but debility lasts for a week or two.

Prevention. In regions where the sandfly is prevalent bed nets must have a fine mesh (forty holes to the linear inch) in order to exclude this very small fly. Since the insect does not fly very high, sleeping on the roof of a house may serve as a protection.

Sandflies breed in damp, dark places and especially among rubbish and in vines and shrubbery. Premises in which repeated cases have occurred may continue to harbor infected sandflies. Such buildings should be avoided or made safe by destroying rubbish and removing broken down walls and shrubbery. Cracks should be filled up, latrines fumigated with sulphur and dark cellars ventilated and white washed. DDT residual spray should be used and animals and fowls kept at a distance from the house.

No specific *treatment* is known for sandfly fever, but symptoms should be treated as they arise. That is, high fever may be relieved by sponging and copious amounts of cool drinks, with aspirin to relieve the pains. When the bite is noticed, it should be painted with tincture of iodine.

Yellow Fever

Yellow fever (Fievre Jaune, Feibre Amarilla, Amaryl) is due to a virus, conveyed by Aedes aegypti mosquitoes. These bite mainly in the daytime but not in bright sun. The disease gets its name from the jaundice which sometimes, but not always, constitutes a prominent symptom. The disease is not wide spread. Small epidemics have occurred in Africa, on the west coast and in the Anglo-Egyptian Sudan. In South America the disease exists in jungle areas.

Symptoms usually begin with shivering, about two to five days after infection. The next day temperature may rise as high as 104°. Severe headache in the forehead or behind the eyes, is accompanied by flushing and swelling of the face, with pains in the back, legs and abdomen. The pulse, although as rapid as 100 beats per minute at first, either remains stationary or falls, and is soft and weak. Jaundice appears in typical cases on about the third day and increases throughout the illness. The enlarged liver can be felt below the ribs on the right side of the abdomen. On the third or fourth day "stage of calm" begins. The temperature falls and other symptoms improve. Then either the patient may proceed to get well, or he may develop fever again, with increasing jaundice, and possible hemorrhage from the stomach or nose.

About 25 per cent of sufferers from yellow fever die, usually on about the sixth day. Some cases are so mild that the patient does not go to bed. It is said that if the initial fever does not exceed 105° chances for recovery are good.

Prevention by vaccination is important. Immunization should be repeated every two years. Measures should be taken against the mosquito. This variety prefers vessels containing water—vases, flower pots, roof gutters, tire casings, etc.—as breeding places.

There is no specific treatment for yellow fever. The patient should remain under a mosquito net. The bowels should be kept open using a dose of Epsom salts at the beginning of symptoms and enemas afterward. Much fluid should be drunk and baking soda in the amount of 1 teaspoonful every 4 hours administered in the fluid. In the early stages citrus fruit juice only should be given as food. Later, light starchy foods may be given, but very little fat.

Kala Azar

Kala azar (visceral leishmaniasis, dum-dum fever, or sahib's disease), which resembles chronic malaria, is characterized by irregular fever, enlargement of the spleen and liver, with bleeding from nose and gums and severe anemia. It is due to a microscopic parasite, (Leishmania), probably conveyed by sandflies. Six weeks to four months after the infecting bite the onset of the disease may be either sudden or gradual, with high fever ushered in by a chill and vomiting. After two to six weeks, the fever may go away only to return later, recurring for months. Profuse sweats are common and later there may be swelling of the ankles and legs. The skin may assume an earthy gray color.

Without specific treatment 90 per cent of patients die within two and one half years. Manson Bahr says: "The outstanding clinical feature which impresses itself on one's mind is that, in spite of the patient's weak and emaciated condition—he preserves a good appetite and a clean tongue, while with a temperature of 102 degrees he may be doing his work and be quite unaware that he has fever. In this respect kala-azar differs from malaria and other toxic fevers such as typhoid."

Intravenous injection of antimony compounds is usually effective in treatment. The "pentavalent" preparations of antimony, including neostibosan and urea stibamine, are now used in preference to the "trivalent" tartar emetic for the purpose.

Relapsing Fever

Relapsing fever (also known as tick fever, louse fever, famine fever, or spirochaetal fever) is the term applied to a group of diseases conveyed by lice or ticks. Louse-borne relapsing fever occurs in parts of Europe and Asia, especially China and North Africa. Tick-borne varieties of the disease are found in Central Africa among other places. The soft tick, responsible for relapsing fever in Central Africa is an oval, rotund, greenish-brown animal which is one-third inch or less in length and has a leathery surface. Its habits are similar to those of bedbugs.

Relapsing fever, in general is characterized by a period of fever lasting two to six days and followed, after apparent recovery, by one or more relapses. Without microscopic examination of the blood for the spirochete causing this disease, diagnosis is difficult. A high, prostrating fever which relapses about fourteen days after the beginning of symptoms, however, is suggestive of relapsing fever.

Prevention is most effectively accomplished by use of DDT in talcum powder applied on the person and on the inside of clothing. Insect repellents are also excellent. Other means for prevention include the avoidance of infected areas such as old camp sites and native houses in places where the disease is prevalent. Bed nets and beds raised above the floor on smooth legs which ticks cannot climb are a protection to the sleeper. Travelers should carry their own camp cots and when putting them up should set the legs in tin cans filled with cresol or other disinfectant solution. A light should be kept burning at night, since ticks swarm when lights are out. Bedding and baggage should be carefully searched before resuming a journey.

As a preventive of the tick-borne disease Chesterman recommends that prophylactic doses of acetarsone (stovarsal) tablets be taken on the first and third day after exposure to tick bites. A dose of 0.25 grams (4 grains) may be taken 5 or 6 times on each of these days. In treatment of the fever, careful nursing with a nutritious liquid diet should be provided. Vitamin C can be added to fruit juice and vitamin B_1 to soup. This diet should be continued after the crisis, even though the patient is ravenously hungry and believes himself well. In specific treatment, penicillin is probably best, and the next best is 2 to 4 intravenous injections of arsphenamines, although these should not be given when crisis is imminent.

For Central African, tick-borne relapsing fever when intravenous injections of arsphenamines are not available acetarsone (stovarsol) tablets may be given by mouth in doses of 0.25 gram (4 grains) 5 or 6 times daily. Chesterman prefers this method of treating the Central African variety, but stovarsol is far from being a harmless drug and may give arsenic poisoning to some patients.

Epidemic Typhus (*True Typhus, Louse Typhus, Jail Fever, Putrid Fever, Petechial Fever, European Typhus*)

Definition. An acute fever, usually of abrupt onset, lasting fourteen days.

Cause. Bacterialike bodies, called Rickettsia, transmitted by the louse.

Distribution. Europe has been the chief center of great typhus epidemics of the world. Such epidemics are sometimes associated with war. The disease has appeared in Asia, Africa and North and South America. It is most frequent in cold weather when heavy clothing and crowding of human beings favor the breeding and transmission of lice.

Symptoms. The patient becomes ill about six to fourteen days after infection, often suffering from headache, backache, nausea and weakness. At the end of the second day or sooner the temperature begins to rise and by the third or fourth day has reached 103° or 104°. Sometimes chills or chilliness precede the fever. The face becomes flushed. Temperature falls rapidly at the end of the second week. Those who die usually do so then. While fever lasts there is great prostration, the mouth is foul, the intellect clouded. Delirium may occur. A *rash* appears on the third to the fifth day. This resembles the rash of measles. It seldom occurs on the face however, but is most marked on the back.

Complications which may develop include broncho-pneumonia and gangrene of the extremities.

Mortality varies in different epidemics. It may be as low as 5 per cent or as high as 70 per cent.

Prevention. Anti-typhus vaccine should be administered in anticipation of exposure and repeated every four to six months. House to house inspection for cases and quarantine of patients in treatment centers should be practiced. DDT sprinkled in the seams of garments is a useful preventive of louse infestation.

Delousing Measures. These include shaving the body, clipping the hair, washing the skin and hair and immediately applying to all hairy parts DDT either as a powder (10 per cent) in talc or as an emulsion in the form of NBIN. The application should be repeated after a week. Clothes should be disinfected. This can be done by steam sterilization or by boiling for five minutes. When this is impracticable, clothing may be soaked in 5 per cent cresol or 2 per cent lysol solution, or treated with 10 per cent DDT in talcum powder.

Storage of clothing for thirty days, in cold weather, or for three weeks in warm weather results in death of lice by starvation.

Those attending patients or carrying out delousing measures should in addition to applying DDT powder to their persons and clothing, wear overalls with wrists and ankles fitted under gloves and boots. The face, and especially the eyes should be protected by masks and goggles from droplet infection. This special garb is very necessary for inspectors, as epidemics may result from contact and inhalation of lice feces.

Treatment. Para-aminobenzoic acid, one of the B-complex vitamins, is coming to be considered as specific for this and other diseases of the typhus group, called "rickettsial diseases." The drug is given by mouth in powder form with an accompanying dose of bicarbonate of soda. An initial dose of 8 grams (2 drams) is followed by 3 grams (45 grains) every 2 hours.

More recently Aureomycin and Chloromycetin have been found effective for typhus fever and other diseases of this group.

Besides specific treatment with para-aminobenzoic acid, good nursing and other measures useful for fevers in general should be provided.

Other Diseases of the Typhus Group (Rickettsial Diseases)

1. Endemic typhus or Murine typhus (Brill's disease), carried by rat fleas.
2. Trench fever, carried by lice.
3. Japanese river fever, carried by mites.
4. Rocky Mountain spotted fever, carried by ticks.
5. South African tick typhus, carried by ticks.
6. Q. fever, carried by ticks.
7. Other types of fever transmitted by ticks or mites.
Treatment. The same as for epidemic typhus.

Undulant Fever (Malta Fever, Mediterranean Fever, Goat Fever, Brucellosis)

Definition. A group of fevers, usually of long duration, associated with weakness, sweating and rheumatic pains.

Cause. Three varieties of Brucella organisms are responsible for the disease in various locations. In Malta where the disease is so common as to be given the name "Malta fever," the germ is conveyed through unpasteurized milk or milk products from infected goats. In the United States some cases result from using unpasteurized milk of cows which are infected with a contagious disease causing abortion in cattle. Another type in the United States is contracted by handling the carcasses of infected swine.

Distribution. Although the disease is best known in Malta and countries of the Mediterranean basin, it can occur anywhere. It is wide spread in the United States and known to occur in the Sudan, South Africa, Somaliland, Northwest India, China, the Philippines, and Mexico. In Malta, the fever begins most often in the summer, soon after the kidding season when milk is heavily infected.

Symptoms. These may begin as early as six days and as late as several months after infection. The patient suffers from headache, sleeplessness, and lack of appetite. Fever may or may

not be ushered in by chill. Fever may be very severe and continuous until death occurs or at the other extreme it may be
intermittent and so mild that the patient, although feeling
miserable does not go to bed. The term "undulant" fever refers to the type of the disease in which fever occurs in waves.
After a week or two of acute illness the temperature falls to
normal only to rise again at the end of a few days in the first
of a long series of relapses. Prominent symptoms are profuse
sweating, constipation, anemia, emaciation and fleeting pains
in the joints. Relapses may continue for three to nine months
or more than a year. Eventually the temperature remains normal but the patient has by this time become a chronic sufferer
from weakness and fatigue so that he may be unable to resume
his work for some time.

Mortality. This is in general about 2 to 6 per cent. A
continued temperature of 104° (40° C.) is an unfavorable
sign.

Diagnosis. The disease is often mistaken for typhoid fever.
Laboratory tests of the blood make diagnosis possible. A skin
test is also available.

Prevention. Most cases of undulant fever could have been
prevented by the simple expedient of pasteurizing or boiling
milk and milk products. The cases which are due to handling
infected carcasses can be prevented by the wearing of long
rubber gloves by those working in packing houses. Protective
inoculation against the disease is possible and should be routine among slaughter house employees and for laboratory
workers whose work includes measures for the diagnosis of
undulant fever.

Treatment. For *acute cases* Chloromycetin is probably the
drug of choice. Aureomycin and streptomycin with sulfadiazine have also given good results. For *chronic cases* no treatment has been found specific. Good nutrition, good hygiene,
and the relief of pain by aspirin exert a beneficial effect.

Sleeping Sickness (*African Human Trypanosomiasis*)

This should not be confused with Encephalitis which is, in
the United States, sometimes called "sleeping sickness."

Definition. An infection occurring in Africa and character-ized by fever, often prolonged and intermittent, weakness and protracted lethargy which may be followed by insanity and death.

Distribution. This disease is found only in tropical Africa.

Cause. Microscopic organisms called trypanosomes (Tryp-anosoma gambiense and Trypanosoma rhodesiense) are trans-mitted by different varieties of tsetse flies. Animals, especially large game but also domestic animals, are thought to become reservoirs of the disease.

Tsetse flies are somber-colored insects, larger than stable flies. Most species bite only in the daytime and are attracted by dark-colored clothes. The bite is usually painless. Those who wear no clothing are most exposed to infection.

These flies are found in circumscribed districts, or belts, usually in shady regions at the side of a stream, on the edge of a forest or sometimes on wooded plains. The larvae develop to maturity in the female fly.

Period Between Infection and the Beginning of Symptoms. This period is three weeks.

Symptoms. 1. *First stage:* The area of the bite becomes in-flamed and painful. Irregular fever, which is not influenced by quinine, may last for weeks. Swelling of the face and of the eyes is sometimes present. A little later lymph glands become swollen especially in the neck and armpits. Itching of the skin and rashes are noticed especially in the case of white patients.

2. *Second stage:* Gradually most of the first-stage symptoms increase. The lymph glands however, are now smaller, and harder. The body becomes swollen and flabby. It is said that not until this second stage do the native Africans, suffering from the disease complain. Those who are noticed to be wear-ing a string around the head or to be using native medicines for headache are usually already in the second stage. In this stage the muscles twitch and the tongue trembles when ex-truded. The sufferer is sluggish mentally. His character de-teriorates and he cannot be trusted. The body becomes dirty

and covered with sores. Eventually the patient becomes drowsy and sometimes maniacal.

3. *Terminal stage:* The sufferer is now emaciated and appears too lazy to speak, move, or eat. He may die in convulsions or in deep unconsciousness.

Mortality. Untreated, the disease is almost invariably fatal. Death occurs after three months to three years of illness. In some districts sleeping sickness has reduced the native population by as much as two-thirds. There is hope for recovery with proper treatment, so long as the patient is able to sit up.

Diagnosis. This can be made by finding the typanosomes in the blood, the spinal fluid or in material withdrawn through a hypodermic needle from the lymph glands. Lay workers recognize the disease by the presence of persistent headache, swollen glands in the neck, and tremor of the tongue.

Prevention. 1. *Personal measures:* When it is necessary to travel in daylight through regions known to be infected, light-colored clothes should be worn, together with veils, gloves and leggings. A preliminary injection of Bayer 205 or Pentamidine should also be taken as a preventive of the disease. The repellent 6–2–2–mixture, mentioned under relapsing fever, should be used.

2. *Public-health measures:*

(*a*) Periodic examination for swollen glands of all inhabitants of infected areas at intervals of six months.

(*b*) Treatment of all those found to be infected.

(*c*) In rapidly spreading epidemics preventive injections of Bayer 205 given to all inhabitants. This protects for three months or more. Mass prophylaxis is also practiced by giving injections of Pentamidine every six months.

(*d*) Restriction of travel to or from infected areas.

(*e*) Clearing away underbrush and trees on watercourses frequented by native Africans. (Carriers on motor roads are likely to become infected.)

(*f*) Evacuation of infected village sites or even whole districts.

(g) Catching tsetse flies with sticky preparations or with fly traps.

Treatment. The earlier treatment is begun the better is the prospect for cure. Two drugs are given by *intravenous injection.* These are Bayer 205 (synonyms: Germanin, Forneau 309, Moranyl and Antrypol) and Tryparsamide. In the *first stage* five injections of Bayer 205 at weekly or shorter intervals may produce a cure. *In cases which have reached the second stage* Tryparsamide is the best drug. It should be preceded, however, by three injections of Bayer 205. A period of two or three weeks should elapse after this preliminary treatment. Then Tryparsamide is injected for 6 to 8 doses at 5-day intervals. Accidents sometimes occur after the use of both of these drugs and injection should be given by a doctor experienced in their use.

Accessory Treatment. Patients are often suffering from several other diseases when infected with trypanosomiasis. For this reason they should be examined especially for hook worm and schistosomiasis and treated for these diseases if indicated, at an early date. A liberal diet is needed and treatment of anemia with iron is often useful.

South American Trypanosomiasis (Chaga's Disease)

This disease, which is rarely encountered, is due to Trypanosoma cruzi. It is transmitted by reduvid (winged) bugs sometimes called "assassin" or "kissing" bugs. Besides the human being, cats, dogs and other animals are susceptible to the disease.

Symptoms are severe in infants under two years of age. In adults the disease may be mild. About ten days after the infecting bite a high, continuous fever begins. Inflammation of one eye and swelling of one side of the face are distinctive signs. The liver, spleen and heart may be affected and the glands enlarged. In the chronic stage serious involvement of the nervous system and the heart occur and dropsy may become general.

Treatment. This is principally symptomatic. Recently

Bayer 7602 given by intramuscular injections has been reported to be beneficial.

Plague (*Pest, Black Death*)

Definition. An acute infectious disease characterized by sudden onset, fever, severe prostration and usually either painful swellings of the glands, called buboes, or more rarely, in the pneumonic type, of pneumonia.

Cause. An organism called the Bacillus pestis, carried by the rat flea. Plague is primarily a disease of rodents, especially rats but also other rodents including the marmot in Siberia, shrews and garbilles in Africa and ground squirrels in California and other Western States. The rats most dangerous to man locally are the black domestic variety, called "Rattus rattus," but the gray Norwegian rat (which occurs in this country) is more responsible for spreading the disease widely. Epidemics occur in the season most favorable to the multiplication of fleas. Extreme heat and dryness are unfavorable to its spread. Circumstances predisposing to the development of plague are filth, poor sanitation which provides rats access to food and harborage, poverty, the existence of former epidemics in the same place, a moderate temperature and a moist atmosphere.

Distribution. Almost world wide. In India plague has caused over a million deaths in a year. It is found also in South China, the Netherlands Indies, Africa, especially in the north, central and southern parts and along the seaboard, parts of South America and a yearly case or two in California in the United States. In London the "Great Plague" occurred in 1665. The disease may be introduced at any port by sick rats or patients, or by infected fleas in bedding or baggage.

Mode of Infection. (a) In *bubonic plague* infection usually takes place through the bite of fleas which have fed on plague-stricken rats or patients. Occasionally, the disease is acquired through infective material which enters the body through cuts or scratches.

(b) In *pneumonic plague* infection occurs through breathing in droplets of sputum from a patient suffering from this disease.

Varieties of Plague.
1. Bubonic type.
2. Pneumonic type.
3. Septicaemic type.
4. Ambulatory type or Pestis Minor.

1. *Bubonic plague:* This is the most common variety, named for the buboes, or swollen infected glands by which it is characterized. Symptoms usually begin three to five days after infection. The onset may be gradual or sudden, with a chill, headache, fever, and prostration. Vomiting may occur. The mind is dull, the speech faltering, the features drawn and the expression either apathetic or anxious. If the patient can walk he staggers like a drunken man. The temperature may be 103° or 104°, reaching 106° or 107° before death. The pulse is very rapid, the skin dry, the face bloated and the eyes sunken or bloodshot. The bowels are usually constipated.

Buboes generally appear within twenty-four hours but may occur at any time from the first few hours to the fifth day. Of these 75 per cent are situated in the groin. Occasionally, and especially in children, buboes are seen in the arm pit or neck. As to size, buboes may be smaller than walnuts or as large as goose eggs. They are painful and tender. The skin over the swellings is red. Pus forms in the buboes and when rupture occurs, extensive sores result. Hemorrhages may occur under the skin. These are called "death tokens." Gangrene may develop on the buttocks, abdomen, limbs, face and other parts.

In severe cases the patient becomes very dull mentally. Delirium, stupor and profound unconsciousness may ensue. Death, in fatal cases, usually occurs between the third and fifth days, from heart failure. In non-fatal cases after buboes appear profuse perspiration occurs and symptoms subside. Buboes enlarge and if not incised finally burst. Sometimes they persist a month before bursting. The pus may have a foul odor. Occasionally buboes are absent. As a rule, convalescence begins between the sixth and tenth days but it may be delayed until after two or three weeks.

2. *Pneumonic plague:* This type, in most epidemics, comprises 3 to 4 per cent of all the cases. In a few epidemics most

of the cases are of the pneumonic type. A low environ-
mental temperature and moist atmosphere are favorable to its
spread.

Symptoms resemble those of pneumonia but are accompanied by greater prostration. The sputum is thin and blood-
stained rather than rusty and sticky, as in pneumonia. No
buboes are present.

3. *Septicaemic plague:* This is a form of blood poisoning. It
is due to an early and overwhelming invasion of the blood
by the plague bacillus and may lead to death without the appearance of either buboes or pneumonia.

4. *Ambulatory plague:* In this type the patient is only
slightly ill and continues to walk about. He may or may not
have buboes.

Mortality: Plague has been considered the most fatal of all
epidemic diseases. In bubonic plague the mortality has aver-
aged in the past, 75 per cent. Now, when treatment of bubonic
plague with sulfa drugs is begun on the first day of illness and
continued for a week or ten days without interruption most
patients will recover. But vaccinated persons who are exposed
and acquire the disease may not survive unless they are adequately treated in this way.

Formerly all cases of pneumonic plague were fatal. With
the use of new drugs a few recoveries have now been reported.
Sulfadiazine, sulfamerazine, and streptomycin have been used
with success.

Means of Prevention. 1. Houses and ships should be rat-
proof. The lower parts of a house should be built of hard brick
or concrete and all vents covered with wire netting. A curtain
wall four inches thick is sunk eighteen inches into the earth all
the way around. This should have a right angle flange, one
inch thick, extending out for eight inches.

2. Rats are prevented from entering or leaving ships by
keeping ships always at least four feet from the wharf, by placing guards and funnels on ropes leading to wharfs and by
taking gangways up when not in use.

3. Rats should be destroyed by means of fumigation, traps
or poison. At times of epidemics a method must be chosen

which will simultaneously kill fleas. Dead rats should be burned.

4. For destroying fleas DDT in 10 per cent dilution in talc dust or discarded flour is probably best. They are also killed by fumigation, or kerosene emulsion.

5. Immunization with anti-plague vaccine, repeated in six months if exposure continues.

6. Isolation of patients for three weeks after complete recovery and quarantine of travelers from infected ports for a period of at least five days. If infection has occurred symptoms will usually show themselves in two to five days.

7. Protection of those who care for plague patients is accomplished by means of

(a) Using a screened ward from which animals (e.g. cats) and fleas are excluded.

(b) Dusting DDT powder on ward floors and especially into the corners.

(c) Undressing patients on a white sheet so as to see any fleas, and after applying DDT putting all the clothes into a bag for sterilization by steam (autoclaving).

(d) Applying DDT powder to the patients themselves.

(e) Using anti-plague vaccine and anti-plague serum injected on the same day and followed, in ten days, by second dose of vaccine.

(f) The wearing of boots and puttees to protect the legs, and overalls closed with elastic at the neck, ankles and wrists.

(g) The wearing of gloves, either of rubber or, for rough work, of chamois to protect from infection through cuts and scratches on the hands.

(h) The daily disinfection of attendants and their clothes.

8. Disposal by burning of excreta and garbage. Bedding, clothes and other articles contaminated by discharges from patients to be sterilized by autoclaving, boiling, or soaking for one hour in 5 per cent cresol or 10 per cent formalin solution.

9. Cremation of the dead with as little delay as possible. If this is impossible they should be buried in deep graves.

10. Disinfection of the house in which the patient was ill

with DDT. Inexpensive houses or even whole villages are
sometimes burned.

Treatment. 1. *Drugs:* Sulfonamides are to be used in huge
doses. Six grams is the initial dose of sulfadiazine. Then 2
grams every 4 hours. Large water intake (3000 to 4000 cc.)
must be maintained, by vein if necessary. An output of 1500 cc.
of urine daily is essential. The above doses are to be continued
until improvement, then gradually reduced, but some of the
sulfa drug should be given for at least 1 week of normal temperature.

2. *Intravenous injection* of anti-plague serum, begun as
soon as possible and repeated every 8 to 10 hours until symptoms abate.

3. *Good nursing:* The patient should be kept in bed until
the temperature has remained normal for three or four days.
The fever should be treated with luke-warm sponges every
hour or two and an ice cap used for headache. Heart stimulants may be needed. Morphine may be given to relieve distress
and promote sleep. A liquid diet is indicated while fever continues and much water should be drunk.

4. *Treatment of buboes:*

(*a*) Painting with tincture of iodine if pus has not formed.

(*b*) The continued application of hot, wet dressings while
buboes are red and painful.

(*c*) The incision of buboes which are "ripe." *Caution:* Do
not incise early.

(*d*) Antiseptic dressings to ruptured or incised buboes.

20

THE DYSENTERIES:
AMOEBIC AND BACILLARY

NEXT TO MALARIA, the greatest disease problems in the tropics and the subtropics in general are the dysenteric diseases. By
this is meant diseases which give rise to loose stools containing
blood and mucus. Although these symptoms are sometimes
associated with other infections the terms "the dysenteries"
is meant to refer only to amoebic and bacillary dysentery.
These two diseases probably constitute the greatest potential
disease hazard associated with travel in tropical parts of the
world. Unfortunately no vaccines have as yet been prepared
to immunize against infections of this kind. All the greater,
for this reason, is the need for education in their regard.

AMOEBIC DYSENTERY (AMOEBIASIS)

Definition

Amoebic dysentery is an infection of the lining of the large
intestine with the microscopic animal parasite, the *entamoeba
histolytica.*

Distribution

The disease may occur anywhere. Even in localities where
it has previously been unknown an infected person may start
an epidemic, usually by infecting the water supply. But amoebic dysentery is more common in the tropics and semitropics
than elsewhere and is especially prevalent in India, Indo-

China, China, the Philippines, North and Central Africa, Central America and South America, the West Indies and the southern part of the United States.

Cause

The cause is infection with the entamoeba histolytica, usually through food or drink contaminated with the faeces of patients or of carriers of the disease.

The entamoeba histolytica, like other amoebae, can alter its shape by throwing out fingerlike projections. In this manner it surrounds and ingests blood cells. Boring its way through the lining of the intestine it can reach the liver and give rise to liver abscess. The lining of the intestine is often riddled with ulcers resulting from its action.

The amoeba in the form described can be found in blood and mucus contained in fresh stools at the beginning of an infection. Later, under certain circumstances, amoebae become smaller, lose their activity and their power of ingesting blood cells and change into "cysts." In formed stools, cysts are to be expected rather than the motile forms. It is these cysts in the stools of infected persons which often contaminate food and drink and give rise to new cases of the disease. The discovery of cysts in the stools of apparently healthy persons establishes their role as carriers. Neither patients suffering from the disease nor carriers should be allowed to handle food. Only by the most scrupulous cleansing of the hands can they avoid contaminating the substances they handle.

Sources of Infection.

1. Contaminated water or ice used in drinks.

2. Contaminated fingers conveying the cysts to food or directly to the mouth.

3. Flies.

4. The contamination of garden produce eaten raw, with human excreta used as fertilizer.

The period between infection and the beginning of symptoms is, as a rule, at least twenty to ninety days or even longer. Occasionally in an epidemic it is as short as seven days.

Chances of recovery are excellent with proper and adequate treatment of the infection in its early stages. Correct treatment is also successful in many chronic cases. Without proper treatment the disease may be the cause of poor health over a period of many years and may finally prove fatal. The final and complete elimination of cysts from the stools of chronic carriers may be difficult to achieve; and many cases which have actually been cured are afterwards reinfected.

Symptoms

Mild Cases. An infected person may be quite unaware that he is ill. He may never have noticed blood or mucus in his stools. At times his chief complaint may concern periods of constipation. For months or even years he may suffer from symptoms of indigestion, vague abdominal discomfort, slight anemia, fatigue and nervous irritability without knowing that these symptoms are due to infection. In persons who have lived where this disease is common any complaint of poor health or lack of strength should be suspected of being due to amoebic dysentery especially if there has been an occasional attack of "loose bowels."

Severe Cases. These sometimes begin suddenly with acute symptoms. They cannot be diagnosed from bacillary dysentery except by laboratory tests. There are frequent discharges containing blood and mucus together with straining, abdominal tenderness, colicky pains, and very occasionally fever and marked prostration. Pieces of the lining of the intestine may be passed with the stools. Death may result from exhaustion, hemorrhage, perforation of the intestine, or from complications, especially liver abscess. In most instances acute symptoms subside and the disease becomes chronic. In chronic amoebic dysentery, while the patient may be in fair health most of the time, chilling of the abdomen, errors of diet or indulgence in alcohol often bring on acute symptoms. Eventually anemia and emaciation may result.

Complications

The chief complication of amoebic dysentery is liver abscess. Occasionally, abscesses occur in the brain, spleen or other organs. Liver abscess may develop in a person who is not conscious of having suffered from dysentery. The collection of pus in the liver, pressing against the diaphragm tends to make breathing painful. There is usually a sense of fulness under the right, lower ribs. An irregular temperature rising in the evening to 103° to 105° and falling to a much lower level in the morning is suggestive of an abscess. Occasionally the abscess perforates the diaphragm and the pus is coughed up as sputum.

Laboratory Diagnosis

The discovery of the entamoeba hystolytica or of cysts of this amoeba in stools establishes the diagnosis. Finding the organisms is sometimes difficult, however, and a negative report from examination does not necessarily rule out the possibility of infection. If a patient suffers from symptoms suggestive of amoebic dysentery and has lived where that disease is common the doctor may think it wise in chronic cases to give treatment for amoebic dysentery even in the presence of negative laboratory findings. But if a doctor and laboratory facilities are available the amoeba is to be found in the stools in acute cases and usually also in chronic infections. It needs to be remembered that bacillary dysentery, mild or severe, acute or chronic, is nine times as common as amoebic dysentery.

Prevention

The boiling of drinking water and the avoidance of contact of ice with drinks has been discussed on page 35. Exclusion of flies from privies, kitchens and dining rooms is another important means of prevention. Where night soil is used as fertilizer no raw fruit or vegetables can safely be eaten without the special preparation described on page 38. Nursing technique to prevent discharges of dysentery patients from spreading infection has been outlined on page 91. Probably the most important single precaution is the habit of always washing the hands before meals and before preparing food and also before leaving the lavatory. The safest food can be infected by the fingers of those who handle it. All those who handle food for the household should have their stools examined once in six months.

Those found to be dysentery carriers should be suspended from contact with food, treated and returned to their former work only when pronounced cured.

Treatment of Amoebic Dysentery

1. *Treatment of Acute Attacks.* The patient should be put to bed and given a liquid diet consisting of clear soup, albumin water, barley water or rice water and weak tea. When diarrhea abates, a semisolid, nourishing diet is indicated, such as that recommended for typhoid fever (on page 155).

Treatment with emetine (derived from ipecac): It is taken for granted that a doctor has seen the patient, had a specimen of the stools examined and diagnosed the case. He will probably inject *emetine hydrochloride* (1 grain or 0.06 gram), once a day, subcutaneously for from 4 to 7 days, preferably only until acute symptoms subside. This treatment requires the service of a physician because of possible ill effects of emetine on the heart. Emetine is the only drug known to kill the amoebae outside, as well as inside, the intestinal tract. Any dysentery that does not improve after two or three doses of emetine is certainly not due to the entamoeba histolytica.

Other drugs, besides emetine, used in the treatment of amoebic dysentery: Carbarsone and drugs of the oxyquinoline sulfonic acid group, including diodoquin, vioform, chiniofon, anayodin and quinoxyl are preferably given in acute cases in addition to emetine injections. One who is not a physician, and for that reason should not administer emetine, can in an emergency give one of these drugs as a substitute. The only known contraindications are disease of the liver or kidney.

Carbarsone: This drug owes its effectiveness to the arsenic contained. Not more than 0.5 gram should be given in a day. *Doses of 0.25 gram should be taken twice a day* for 10 days.

Vioform: Of this, 0.75 gram may be given in a day. It is recommended in doses of 0.25 gram 3 times a day for a week.

Chiniofon (or "Yatren"): Three grams of chiniofon may be given by physicians in 24 hours. The unqualified worker should give only 0.5 gram three times a day, after meals, for 7 days. If chiniofon produces diarrhea or abdominal discom-

fort these effects can be offset by giving small doses of paregoric, e.g. ½ to 1 teaspoonful for an adult or five drops to a
child of one year (see page 261).

Doses of *anayodin* and *quinoxyl* are the same as those of
chiniofon. These drugs of the oxyquinoline sulfonic acid
group kill amoebae in the intestinal contents but not those
which have entered tissues such as the liver.

2. *Treatment of Carriers of Amoebic Dysentery.* By the
term "carriers" is meant persons who are not acutely ill but
have cysts in their stools which might give rise to the infection
of other people. The symptomless or relatively symptomless
cyst-passers may often be effectively treated by carbarsone
alone. Doctors may give 3 or 4 capsules, each 0.25 gram (4
grains) by mouth 3 times a day for 7 to 10 days. Unqualified
workers had better restrict themselves to the doses already
mentioned, i.e. 0.25 gram twice a day for 10 days. Rare toxic
symptoms which may follow the use of this drug include abdominal distress, nausea, vomiting, and a skin eruption. Stools
should, whenever possible, be re-examined 4 to 6 weeks after
treatment, and again at the end of 3 months.

Chiniofon is often used for treatment of cyst-passers. It may
be used in the doses already given (0.5 gram 3 times a day, after
meals, for 7 days). It is recommended that a second course of
treatment, with carbarsone, should follow after an intermis-
sion of a week.

The wearing of a light woolen band in order to prevent
chilling of the abdomen is useful in preventing attacks of diarrhea in those who have suffered from chronic amoebic dysentery. This measure may be needed only when sleeping out of
doors.

Treatment of liver abscess and other amoebic abscesses: The
injection of emetine is, as a rule, successful. Emetine may be
given by a physician in doses of 0.06 gram daily by injection,
for 8 to 10 days to patients with amoebic liver abscess. This
treatment should not be repeated for at least 3 weeks. In other
cases the doctor may withdraw pus by means of a large needle
attached to a syringe. Surgical operation is seldom necessary.

BACILLARY DYSENTERY (EPIDEMIC DYSENTERY)

Definition

Bacillary dysentery is an acute epidemic disease due to infection of the lining of the large intestine by various species of the organism, Shigella dysenteriae.

Distribution

This disease is about nine times as common as amoebic dysentery. It is found throughout the world but is especially prevalent and severe in the tropics and semitropics. Conditions of crowding are favorable to the spread of the disease in asylums, prison camps and military barracks.

Cause

The cause is usually contamination of food or drink with the faeces of patients or carriers. Unsafe water or ice, uncooked fruits or vegetables and flies may convey the infection. Diapers of babies suffering from dysentery should not be exposed to flies. In hospitals unsterilized bedpans and enema equipment may spread the disease from patient to patient.

The period between infection and the beginning of symptoms is short, usually one to seven days.

Mortality in well-nourished individuals is seldom higher than 5 per cent although some cases are quickly fatal. Among the poorly nourished of the native population the mortality in some epidemics may be 40 to 50 per cent. *Complication with malaria greatly increases danger from the disease.*

Symptoms

The onset is usually abrupt, with diarrhea and colicky pains. Blood and mucus appear in the stools. Eventually the stools consist of little besides blood and mucus. The abdomen is tender on pressure. Straining at stool may be very painful and eventually the lining of the rectum may be pushed out and continue to protrude. Stools are small in amount and not very offensive.

Some cases are so mild as not to be recognized as dysentery

while in other cases stools may number ten to thirty or even sixty in a day. The temperature often rises to 101° to 103°. Rarely there may be muscular pains, headache, delirium and stupor. Vomiting is common but not persistent.

Mild cases yield to treatment promptly. In others the disease may last several weeks. Very severe infections may be fatal in a few days. Although the disease seldom becomes chronic 3 per cent of cases are said to be carriers. Carriers are usually infectious for not longer than nine months.

Complications

Arthritis is the most common complication. The usual complaint is "rheumatism" in the joints. It often occurs during convalescence and may last for some time but usually disappears eventually leaving no permanent ill effects. In very severe cases perforation of the bowel and peritonitis may occur. Acute inflammation in the eye is another possible complication. *Diagnosis* should, whenever possible, be made by laboratory examination of the stools. A fresh stool preferably containing mucus and blood should be placed in a closed glass jar to give the doctor when he arrives. Apart from laboratory examination the following chart adapted from Manson-Bahr may be of use in diagnosis.

COMPARISON BETWEEN AMOEBIC AND BACILLARY DYSENTERY

Amoebic, "Walking dysentery"	*Bacillary, "Lying-down dysentery"*
1. Onset usually insidious.	1. Onset usually acute.
2. Incubation period [1] long, (20–90 days or more).	2. Incubation period short (7 days or less).
3. Fever rare (unless complicated).	3. Fever common.
4. Duration of the disease may be long: months or years.	4. Duration is usually only days or weeks.
5. Stools are moderately frequent and consist of faeces	5. Stools are very frequent, scanty and odorless. They

[1] The incubation period is the period between infection and the appearance of symptoms.

mingled with mucus and blood; their color is greenish or brownish, "resembling anchovy sauce"; the odor is offensive.

consist mostly of gelatinous blood and mucus, resembling red currant jelly.

6. Straining at stool is not accentuated.

6. Straining is very severe.

7. Stools, tested with litmus paper have an acid reaction.

7. The reaction is alkaline.

8. Complication: abscess, usually in the liver.

8. Complications: arthritis or inflammation of the eye.

9. The disease is endemic (i.e. always present in the locality).

9. There is a tendency to epidemic spread.

Prevention

This is the same as in the case of amoebic dysentery except that chlorinization will kill all the organisms responsible for bacillary dysentery.

Treatment

Immediate and complete rest in bed is indicated. The patient should be kept comfortably warm. A light band about the abdomen may lessen abdominal discomfort. Very ill patients should not get out of bed. If movements become extremely frequent it may be well to dispense with the bed pan and use a pad made of old, soft muslin. Absorbent cotton may be placed within the muslin to catch the blood and mucus which, in severe cases, is expelled almost continuously. The skin of parts irritated by the discharge should be kept clean and covered with a light coating of vaseline. When giving this care the nurse should wear rubber gloves if possible, or at least scrub and disinfect her hands very carefully after contact with discharges. If the lining of the rectum has been extruded by straining and appears as a shiny red tumor in the region of the anus, the protruding mass should be anointed with vaseline and pushed back inside the opening, cupping the fingers in such a way as to return first the part which came out last. Then the anus should be covered with a piece of gauze spread with vaseline, and the buttocks strapped together with adhesive tape outside the area of irritated skin. Such strapping discourages further prolapse of the bowel without interfering with bowel movements.

Food for the first twenty-four hours should consist of clear fluids such as clear broth and, for adults, tea with plenty of sugar. *No milk should be given since milk is said to be not well borne in bacillary dysentery.* The second twenty-four hours, smooth cereal like cream of wheat or rice water or strained oatmeal may be given *without milk.* Barley gruel is also useful or a little rice boiled very soft may be served in broth. When the stools have decreased in number a little meat juice may be expressed from freshly broiled steak and added to rice. If this agrees with the patient he may now have a small amount of tender beef or lamb, ground fine and pan-broiled with a little water. Fruit juice diluted with water and sipped after meals may be given cautiously watching that it does not increase the number of bowel movements. Scraped apple is very useful, if available. Later, as the patient improves he may have a tender, broiled lamb chop, strained spinach, and toast. It should be endeavored to give a well-balanced diet including the needed vitamins. Instead of milk, soybean milk may be used. Food should be given warm and in small quantities, at frequent intervals. When blood and mucus have disappeared from the stools soft boiled eggs, oysters, custards and chicken are useful. Return to the normal diet should be gradual. Fruits and vegetables are the last to be added and anything with seeds, strings or skins should be avoided for several weeks.

Medication. Whenever possible this should be prescribed by a physician. A Shiga bacillus antiserum is available for injection in large doses. This may be effective if used very early in the course of severe infections with Shiga organisms. Bacteriophage is another substance which sometimes gives good results. But although these and other remedies may be indicated in certain cases the use of the sulfa drugs has now become the preferred method of treatment.

Sulfonamides ("sulfa drugs") in Treatment of Bacillary Dysentery. Sulfadiazine is usually the drug of choice. Others of the same group of remedies which have been used include sulfathiazole, sulfapyridine, sulfasuccidine (sometimes spelled sulfasuxidine) and sulfaguanidine.

Sulfadiazine in treatment of bacillary dysentery: An initial dose of 2 grams (4 tablets of 0.5 gram) should be followed by 1 gram every 6 hours for about 6 days. Doses for infants and children are: up to 6 months, ¼ tablet 4 times a day; from 6 months to 1 year, ½ tablet 4 times a day; and an additional quarter tablet for each additional 3 years of age up to 16 years.

Sulfasuccidine: If the patient does not respond to sulfadiazine, treatment may be shifted to the use of sulfasuccidine in doses of 5 grams every 6 hours.

When using these sulfa drugs it is important to give abundant fluids. It is estimated that in order to protect the kidneys from ill effect an adult should take 3500 cc. (about 14 eight-ounce glasses or 7 pints) of fluid. The output of urine should be 1500 cc. (about 3 pints). The urine should be kept alkaline by administering half a teaspoonful of bicarbonate of soda three times a day.

Sulfadiazine as a Preventive Measure. In case of an epidemic of bacillary dysentery one tablet of sulfadiazine (0.5 gram) may be taken by healthy persons twice a day as a preventive of infection. Even with this small dose attention should be paid to an increased intake of fluid.

Saline Treatment. The results of giving sodium sulphate to sufferers from bacillary dysentery are sometimes only slightly less miraculous than those following the sulfa drugs. Anyone could administer this treatment. If sodium sulphate is not available, magnesium sulphate (i.e. Epsom salt) can be substituted, although it is not so good. The dose of sodium sulphate depends upon whether the crystalline or the more concentrated, powdered form is used. Using the powdered form ½ teaspoonful dissolved in a little hot water is taken, before food, from 4 to 8 times a day. The dose is gradually decreased. In the case of the coarser, crystalline salt, the dose is 1 teaspoonful.

For children, the saline treatment may be used, dissolving the dose proportionate to the age [2] in 3 teaspoonfuls of water and giving this in teaspoon doses at intervals of 1 or 2 hours during the day.

Advice for Emergencies. The assistance of a physician is always needed for the care of patients suffering from dysentery. In places where medical care is not always available, however, the lay person should not be entirely helpless in dealing with emergencies of this kind. It is recommended that travelers, destined for the tropics and likely to be left at some time to their own resources, provide themselves with effective medicines for the treatment of both amoebic and bacillary dysentery. A supply of tablets of carbarsone or diodoquin for amoebic dysentery and of sulfadiazine tablets for bacillary dysentery is suggested. But how shall the untrained person know in any given instance whether to use these drugs? And if he thinks one of these remedies is urgently needed how can he diagnose the case and know which one to use?

For the help of anyone who must take upon himself the responsibility for these important decisions the following suggestions are offered:

Diarrhea (no blood in the stools)

The first thing which occurs to the mind of the average person in explanation of a sudden attack of loose bowels is that some indigestible food has been eaten. In slight cases the only measure necessary is to cut out fruits and vegetables from the diet and continue to exclude them until the movements have been normal for several days. In case diarrhea is severe and painful something poisonous may have been eaten. This is evidently the right diagnosis when several people who have eaten the same food develop symptoms simultaneously. The thing to do then is to take a dose of castor oil. Before administering any laxative, however, take the precaution of pressing with the hand on all parts of the abdomen, and especially on

[2] Young's rule for finding the proportionate dose for children of given age is as follows. Divide the child's age by the age plus 12. Thus, for a child of four $\frac{4}{4+12} = \frac{1}{4}$ of the adult dose.

the right side below the level of the umbilicus where the appendix is usually located. Should any spot be found which is so tender that the patient flinches when pressure is made upon it neither castor oil nor any other laxative medicine should be used.

In any event, rest in bed and a diet of weak tea and clear soup are indicated. The abdomen should be kept warmly covered. Most cases of "gyppie tummy," a painful type of diarrhea which is very common in Egypt, will respond to this treatment. On the other hand they are usually made worse by taking milk. When symptoms persist more than a day or two a doctor should always be called. He may find that the case is really one of bacillary or amoebic dysentery.

In many instances of diarrhea the action of castor oil together with rest in bed and a liquid diet will be all that is needed to put an end to an attack. After the intestines have been cleared with castor oil colicky pains usually cease. If they persist relief can usually be secured by taking small doses of paregoric.

Should the diarrhea become somewhat chronic a useful remedy is *kaolin,* in doses of ¼ teaspoonful to 2 teaspoonfuls, according to the severity of the case. The kaolin is to be stirred into a cup of water and repeated every 4 hours until diarrhea ceases. Another effective drug is bismuth subnitrate, given in doses of ¼ to ½ teaspoonful, with a little water, every 4 hours. Bismuth imparts a black color to the stools.

Diarrhea Due to Chronic Amoebic Dysentery. Individuals who have lived where amoebic dysentery is common and have been known to suffer from that disease must always suspect that attacks of diarrhea are due to relapses. It is quite possible that they still harbor amoebae in their intestines. Such persons should ask their physicians what drug to take with them on a journey in case attacks occur when no medical help is available. It may be that they will be advised to take carbarsone. If diarrhea persists after the usual treatment with castor oil, rest and diet they should resort to the medicine for amoebic dysentery whether or not blood appears in the stools.

Severe Attacks of Bloody Diarrhea. When symptoms of

dysentery appear suddenly and the patient is acutely ill with frequent stools containing blood and mucus, bacillary dysentery should always be suspected. Although some cases of amoebic dysentery are of this description, the chances are nine to one in favor of bacillary dysentery. The presence of fever and of painful straining at the time of bowel movements makes the latter diagnosis even more probable. Since the greater immediate danger to life is usually due to the bacillary type of dysentery it is urgent to treat for this disease without delay. It is to be hoped that the traveler dependent on his own resources has packed a supply of sulfadiazine tablets in his kit. If that has not been done perhaps he can administer saline treatment. If his diagnosis has been wrong, since amoebic dysentery is *usually* a chronic disease rather than a quick killing infection, it can be hoped that a doctor may be found in time to give the patient emetine injections, or failing this, that carbarsone, diodoquin or vioform can be given a trial.

In malarial districts never forget malaria. Once more, mention should be made of malaria. Some of the most serious cases in which symptoms of dysentery occur are either due to, or complicated by, infection with malaria. For dangerously ill patients who fail to respond to other treatment it will do no harm to try antimalaria drugs. Success may reward this treatment when every other measure has failed.

21

INTESTINAL DISEASES
OTHER THAN THE DYSENTERIES

᠁᠁᠁᠁᠁᠁᠁᠁᠁᠁᠁᠁᠁᠁᠁᠁᠁

CHOLERA (ASIATIC CHOLERA)

Definition

Cholera is an infectious, epidemic disease characterized by profuse diarrheal discharges of the so-called "rice water" character together with vomiting, painful cramps in the muscles, suppression of urine and collapse.

Distribution

The disease exists continuously in Asia, especially in India. Great epidemics have spread from India through Asia Minor, Egypt, Russia, Central Europe and North and South America.

Cause

The disease is caused by infection with the "Comma bacillus" (Vibrio cholerae).

Circumstances favoring spread of cholera are defective sanitation and crowding. At the time of an epidemic however, all Europeans as well as the native inhabitants are in great danger.

Mode of Transmission

The disease is spread through food and drink contaminated by the stools of patients suffering from cholera. Flies or contaminated objects also may convey the infection. Unsafe water, raw milk and fruits and vegetables eaten raw are especially dangerous.

The period between infection and the beginning of symptoms is usually three to six days, but may be as short as a few hours (or occasionally as long as ten days). Five days is the usual quarantine period to insure that a patient is not in the incubation period. For carriers, either those who are recovering from an attack or those who have manifested no symptoms, two weeks is adequate as the organism dies out rapidly.

Symptoms

These will be considered in four stages.

1. *The Premonitory Stage.* In some cases premonitory symptoms such as diarrhea, languor, depression, nausea and discomfort in the region of the stomach are noticed before cholera is recognized. In other cases there is no premonitory stage but rather a person in excellent health is seized suddenly and without warning with violent symptoms and dies within a few hours.

2. *The Evacuation Stage.* Profuse watery stools are passed one after another, usually without pain. Discharges occur in enormous quantities and are brown at first but later colorless, resembling the water in which rice has been cooked. Vomiting is profuse and the material vomited soon consists of this same "rice water." Vomiting is not associated with nausea and causes little distress. Other symptoms during this stage are great thirst, restlessness and agonizing cramps in the muscles of the abdomen and limbs.

3. *The "Collapse" or "Algid" Stage.* The surface of the body has now become cold and covered with clammy sweat. Even the breath is cold. The temperature, taken in the armpit, may be several degrees below normal although rectal temperature is sometimes higher than normal. The eyes are sunken, the nose looks pinched and the cheeks are hollow. The pulse is difficult to feel. The voice is lost. The patient appears indifferent to what goes on around him but his mind is clear. The urine becomes suppressed.

Possible terminations of this stage are:

(*a*) Death. Usually between five to twenty hours after the beginning of symptoms.

(*b*) Rapid recovery. In such a case the temperature rises to or above normal, urine is voided and the pulse becomes sufficiently strong to be felt at the wrist.

4. *The Stage of Reaction.* Fever occurs and may last only a few hours or be continued as in typhoid fever. Complications such as suppression of urine or pneumonia may now be the cause of death.

Occasional symptoms of cholera include a very high temperature which may register 107° in the arm pit or 109° in the rectum. Pregnant women usually miscarry during or after an attack of cholera.

After effects of cholera include anemia, mental and physical debility, insomnia, fever, ulceration of the cornea of the eye, jaundice, bedsores and gangrene of the feet.

Atypical Varieties of Cholera

1. The *ambulatory* form, in which patients are mildly affected but may serve as carriers of the disease.

2. *"Cholerine"* or "choleraic diarrhea," in which diarrhea is severe but other symptoms are mild.

3. *Very severe cases* ending in death in less than three hours.

4. *"Dry cholera,"* in which poisoning from the cholera germs is so intense that death occurs before there has been any diarrhea.

Mortality

Mortality ranges from 20 to 90 per cent with an average of 50 per cent. Some epidemics are very deadly while others are mild. The very old, the very young and the debilitated have a poorer chance for recovery than other patients.

Diagnosis

At the beginning of an epidemic diagnosis is confirmed by laboratory methods. Later, after the epidemic is known to be in progress, diagnosis is easy. Manson-Bahr suggests that "epidemic diarrhea with a mortality of over 50 per cent may be taken to be cholera." Also any epidemic diarrhea in which patients cease to void urine and lose their ability to speak aloud is likely to be cholera.

Preventive Measures

1. *Quarantine.* This is difficult to execute. The ideal precaution is to examine the stools of all persons entering ports from cholera districts and to isolate both patients and carriers.

2. *Other Public-Health Measures.*

(*a*) Protection of water used for drinking or bathing:

(1) By adding chloride of lime, using for an average-size well 2 glasses of lime dissolved in a pail of water and strained through muslin;

(2) Or by adding potassium permanganate crystals to the well water in the proportion of 60 grains (4 grams) of potassium permanganate to the gallon of estimated capacity. The water should be left until it becomes colorless before being used. Vegetation and anything else which the water contains should be removed before the drug is added.

(3) Buckets should be disinfected with chlorine before being used to draw water from wells.

(*b*) Isolation of the sick in screened rooms and thorough disinfection of their stools and all contaminated bedding and clothing by soaking for at least one hour in 10 per cent formalin or 5 per cent cresol solutions, added in amount equal to the stool or urine.

(*c*) Discovery of carriers among the local population by laboratory examination of stools of persons in contact with the sick and segregation of these people until tests prove their stools to be harmless. If laboratory facilities are not available such people should be segregated for two weeks.

(*d*) Rigid supervision of over-crowded districts to prevent cases being hidden.

(*e*) Campaigns for dissemination of information about the nature and prevention of cholera. This is done by means of literature, posters, parades of illustrative floats and exhibits of various kinds.

(*f*) Vigorous anti-fly campaigns.

(g) Immunization with cholera vaccine. Those entering cholera districts as well as those already living in such places should be thus protected. Revaccination should be practiced every three months while the danger lasts and annually prior to the cholera season.

3. *Personal Prophylaxis.*

(a) Avoid uncooked food or drink. *Hot foods and hot drinks are safest* because food materials may be infected *after* cooking. Protect all foods from flies. Such foods as raw lettuce and celery are especially dangerous. Fruits with heavy peels, like oranges and bananas can be made safe by covering them with boiling water for three to five minutes and then removing the skins. Contaminated fish placed on the ice may infect butter and other foods in the icebox. Ice itself may be made of unsafe water.

(b) Restrict the diet to bland and easily digested foods. Digestive upsets predispose to cholera. Avoid taking medicine, especially purgatives such as Epsom salts unless prescribed by a doctor.

(c) Use no unboiled water for drinking, brushing the teeth, or for finger bowls. When water cannot be trusted, hot tea is a useful substitute. In emergencies chemical disinfection of water (see page 36) is a second choice.

(d) Always wash the hands before eating and before preparing food.

(e) Avoid visiting cholera districts if possible. Newcomers are especially susceptible.

(f) Avoid over-fatigue, undue excitement and exposure to cold and wet. Seek treatment promptly for all digestive disorders. If diarrhea occurs seek medical advice at once. It is said that those receiving sulfadiazine and intravenous injection of blood plasma at the onset of the disease are sure to recover.

Treatment

1. Put the patient to bed, raising the foot of the bed on bricks or blocks. Keep him warm and dry by wiping the skin with hot, dry cloths. Arrange a bed pan comfortably for con-

tinuous use and keep it warm with hot water bottles. Cramps in the legs are best relieved by the intravenous injection of fluids.

2. Give no food while the diarrhea is active. Sips of ice water or soda water may be given for thirst. Larger amounts are likely to be vomited. After diarrhea subsides begin nourishment very cautiously using barley water or rice water. *Do not give milk, broths or jellies.* After three or four days smooth cereal such as cream of wheat or strained oatmeal may be used. Until urine is passed freely no further addition to the diet should be made.

3. Never administer cathartics.

4. *It is very urgent to secure a doctor who can administer intravenous injections.* He will probably inject normal saline solution, alkaline solutions, and perhaps glucose solution to which vitamins are added. After dehydration is relieved, plasma or whole blood may also be injected. *Intravenous injections are the most important measure for saving life.*

5. The doctor will probably administer some sulfa drug. In emergencies, when no doctor can be secured sulfadiazine should be started as early as possible according to directions on page 100, if the patient can retain it.

6. To combat suppression of urine when no doctor can be secured to give injections cloths wrung out of hot water may be applied over the part of the back between the lowest ribs and the hip bones.

7. Nursing precautions. All discharges and soiled linen must be immediately disinfected as just described under "public-health measures." "You can eat cholera, you can drink cholera, but you cannot catch it." You are safe even in a cholera ward if you don't eat, drink or smoke while there and clean up properly after leaving.

SPRUE

SPRUE (also known as tropical diarrhea, Ceylon sore mouth, psilosis) is a chronic diarrheal disease characterized by a very severe form of inflammation of the lining of the digestive tract.

Distribution

Sprue is common in Europeans who live, or have lived in South China, India, Ceylon, the Philippines, Mauritius and Northern Australia. It is found also in Central Asia, the West Indies, Central and South America and the Southern part of the United States. It is rarely seen in North Africa, Palestine and Syria and is apparently absent from Central Africa. Although nationals of countries where the disease occurs are less likely to contract sprue than are Europeans they are not exempt.

Cause

The initial cause of sprue is still unknown. One important factor in the production of the disease is deficiency of vitamins of the B-complex, due either to lack of these vitamins in the diet or to inability of the individual to absorb them.

Prevention

Although knowledge of the cause of sprue is incomplete certain measures are of value in resisting the disease. A well-balanced diet containing milk, meat, eggs, whole cereals, fruits, vegetables constitutes an important safeguard. An excess of starchy foods is to be avoided. Good personal hygiene, including exercise in the open air and plenty of rest and sleep are useful in keeping the digestive process normal. Digestive disorders and dysentery in particular predispose to the disease. Such conditions should receive prompt medical attention.

Symptoms

1. *Sore Mouth.* This is often the first symptom noticed. The tongue and the lining of the mouth become sensitive. Ulcers often appear on the edge or tip of the tongue. Later, the tongue becomes red, bare and glazed or fissured. Soreness may be so great as to prevent eating.

2. *Diarrhea and Abdominal Discomfort.* Diarrhea is characteristic. It occurs in the early morning and consists of large,

pale, frothy stools which have an offensive odor. There may be burning pain in the stomach and the abdomen may be greatly distended with gas.

3. *Anemia.* Under the microscope the blood shows a characteristic anemia, similar to that of pernicious anemia.

4. *Weakness, depression and a muddy discoloration of the skin* may ensue. In extreme cases the patient may lose half his normal weight.

The outlook in mild cases is good, *on condition* that proper and adequate treatment is given. Even in severe and long-standing cases the response to treatment may be gratifying, especially if the patient leaves the tropics. Relapses may be precipitated by either extremely hot or extremely cold climates.

Without adequate treatment, severe cases are usually fatal within a period of one to fifteen years.

Treatment

1. *Liver Extract.* The injection of *crude* liver extract is most important. Injections are given daily or on alternate days for 5 to 15 doses. After this the liver extract is injected at weekly intervals during convalescence. Patients returning to the tropics may require injections twice a month for the rest of their lives. The continuance of treatment is of course a matter for the judgment of the individual physician. Liver extract taken by mouth is inadequate to cure the disease although it may improve the symptoms.

2. *Folic Acid* has recently been used with success for treating the anemia of sprue. Twenty milligrams are given daily.

3. *Nicotinic Acid.* Manson-Bahr advises giving this vitamin in pure form in the amount of 0.150 gram (2.3 grains) daily for six months, in addition to liver injections.

4. *Diet.* A bland, nonirritating diet rich in protein and vitamins and containing little of carbohydrate and fat is indicated for patients suffering from sprue. At the beginning of treatment of severe cases a diet of ground raw meat and milk is prescribed by some physicians. Bananas and strawberries are also beneficial foods. The doctor may, in certain cases, supple-

ment the diet with iron, calcium and vitamin D in medical form.

5. *Auxiliary Treatment.* In severe, long standing cases there is need for

(*a*) Rest: This is best obtained in a hospital.

(*b*) Warmth: Chilling must be avoided. Patients should not be removed from the tropics while the diarrhea is active and should not move to a cold climate until treatment has built up their resistance.

(*c*) Complications, such as malaria or amoebic dysentery, should be recognized and treated.

(*d*) Mental and physical fatigue and pregnancy are conditions which should be avoided since they may bring on relapses.

HILL DIARRHEA

Definition

A form of diarrhea closely resembling that of sprue, which occurs principally in Europeans who go to a cool climate in the hills after residing in the hot lowlands of tropical countries.

Symptoms

After reaching the hills a person who has previously been in good health begins to have diarrhea in the early morning hours, probably between 3 and 5 A.M. Usually one to six stools are passed before 11 A.M. The discharges have an offensive odor and are copious, liquid, pale and frothy. Occasionally, typical sprue may develop.

Treatment

In some cases rest in bed and a liquid diet bring about a cessation of symptoms. Cases which persist in spite of these measures should be treated as sprue.

INTESTINAL WORMS

INFESTATION with intestinal parasites is common in the tropics. The following worms are chosen for description because of their comparative importance.

Round Worm Infestation (*Ascariasis*)

The round worm (Ascaris lumbricoides), is a pinkish gray, translucent worm about the diameter of a goose quill, 6 to 9 inches in length and pointed at both ends. Its incidence is world-wide.

Mode of Infection. Human beings become infected by swallowing the eggs of worms. In places where there is no proper disposal of sewage the eggs discharged in faeces are eventually blown about in the air and may be swallowed with food and drink. In other cases flies may ingest the eggs and later deposit them on food. Sometimes eggs of intestinal worms are taken into the body on vegetables which have been manured with human excreta.

Prevention. The proper disposal of night soil is a most important measure in this respect. The exclusion of flies from kitchens and dining rooms and the careful preparation of food and drink (as described on pages 38–39) are essential.

The Life-History of Round Worms. The female worm in the intestine of a human being discharges eggs in enormous numbers. These require a short period of maturation outside the body before becoming infective. Upon being ingested by human being, after maturation, the eggs hatch out. The embryos which emerge do not settle down at once in the intestine but migrate to the liver and lungs before they finally return to the intestine via the trachea and the esophagus. Becoming mature, the parasites make their abode in the intestine but may take occasional trips into the stomach and even emerge through the mouth or nose. Rarely, asphyxiation may result from obstruction of the larynx, or the worm may enter the eustachian tube which leads from the throat to the ear. It may also carry infection into the bile ducts, with serious effects. Hundreds of worms, matted together, may form an obstructing mass in the intestine.

Symptoms. Usually the patient is not conscious of any symptoms. Frequently, however, there is pain in the region of the navel and discomfort in the stomach. In children, nervous symptoms are common such as fretfulness, ill temper, bad dreams and bed-wetting. When large numbers of worms are present children become pale and pasty-looking. They often have large abdomens and, in extreme cases, appear emaciated.

Diagnosis. This presents no difficulty when worms are seen in the stools. Otherwise microscopic examination reveals eggs of the worms in the faeces.

Treatment. Although santonin and oil of chenopodium have long been favorite remedies for round worm infestation their administration is not free from danger of ill effects. The safest remedy is hexylresorcinal. This is also the most efficient drug and kills pin worms and hook worms which may infest the same patient. The drug is not poisonous and can safely be used for the young, the debilitated and, when necessary, for the pregnant.

As in the case of other treatment for worms, it is advisable for the patient to eat little food on the day before taking hexylresorcinal. Rice and tender meat may be eaten but fibrous vegetables are to be avoided because they protect the parasite from the effect of the drug. Epsom salts (1 or 2 tablespoonfuls for an adult) should be administered at bedtime. Early the following morning hexylresorcinal is to be given on an empty stomach. *The dose* for adults is 1 gram (15 grains). For a child the dose may be estimated by allowing 0.1 gram (1½ grains) for each year of the child's age up to ten years. After ten years, the adult dose is indicated.

Hexylresorcinal must never be given in liquid form or in uncoated pills. Pills must never be chewed, or burning of the mouth will result. Specially coated "crystoids" are available on the market but in their absence sugar-coated pills may be used.

After taking hexylresorcinal the patient may go about his work as usual. He may drink water but should eat nothing for five hours. The next morning he should take another dose of Epsom salts to help expel the worms.

Pin Worm Infestation (*Oxyuriasis*)

The pin worm (thread worm or seat worm) is known as the Oxyuris vermicularis. It is a thread-like worm about one-third to one-half inch in length. Children everywhere are subject to infestation with these worms. Adults in the same families often harbor the parasites.

Mode of Infection. Pin worms lay their eggs in the lowest part of the bowel or even on the skin outside the anus. These eggs lodge under the finger nails during the act of scratching. Eggs are conveyed by the fingers to food or directly to the mouth. Sometimes flies ingest them and deposit them on food. These eggs are infective at once without a period of maturation.

Symptoms. Intense itching about the anus at night is due to the out-wandering of female worms to lay their eggs. An irritated condition of the skin around the anus may result from scratching. Nervous disturbances such as restlessness during sleep, grinding of teeth or picking of the nose are well-known symptoms. Rarely, worms find their way inside the appendix and give rise to appendicitis.

Diagnosis. Worms may be seen in the stools or sometimes on the skin outside the anus. The eggs are hard to find microscopically in the faeces. The best way to secure them for examination is to apply a glass slide first to one side of the anus and then to the other side. This should be done before the morning bath and with the patient bent over and straining slightly.

Treatment. This requires thoroughness and perseverance. Upon discovery of a case of infestation every member of the patient's family should have an examination. Those found to be infected should receive treatment. Otherwise, after being cured the patient may be reinfected by the untreated members of the family. Gentian violet is now considered the best drug for treatment of pin worm infestation. *The dose for a child* is 1 tablet containing ½ grain (0.03 gram) of gentian violet after each meal for eight days. It is preferable to use tablets which are especially coated to prevent their solution before reaching the intestine. *The dose for an adult* is 1 grain (0.06 gram).

One method of administering gentian violet is to give the appropriate dose twice daily, after meals, for 8 days and afterward rest from the medicine for 8 days before repeating the course. Then, after a second rest period of 8 days a third 8-day course of gentian violet is given.

Something can be done for a patient suffering from pin worms even if no medicine can be given by mouth. A daily enema of salt solution, in the strength of a teaspoon of salt to a pint of warm water, is useful for washing worms out of the rectum. Anointing the skin around the anus with mecurial ointment will kill the worms when they wander out at night. The wearing of pajamas instead of nightgowns prevents fingers from becoming infected. The hands and the region around the anus should be washed with soap and water after each movement of the bowels. Soiled bed linen should be sterilized by boiling.

Tape Worm Infestation (Taeniasis)

Tape worms are so named because they are flat, like tape. Some of them look like strings of oblong tickets, fastened together. Each segment is complete in itself, possessing both male and female elements. The head which is smaller than the other segments is furnished with suckers and sometimes hooks, by which it clings to the wall of the intestine. If, after the use of worm medicine, the head is still left in the intestine the worm will form again.

Man is infected with the *"beef tape worm"* (Taenia saginata), especially common in Abyssinia, by eating undercooked, infected beef containing larvae of the worm. Each larva is enclosed in a tiny bladder, or "cystocercus." About two months after the meat containing larvae has been eaten adult worms make their appearance in the human intestine. Eggs of these worms are discharged in faeces and afterward infect the ox or cow when eaten with grass.

Man becomes infected with the *"pork tape worm"* (Taenia solium) as the result of eating undercooked "measly" pork, containing cystocerci. The worm may occur wherever pork is eaten. The pig, in turn, acquires the larval stage of the parasite by eating segments of the adult worm passed in the faeces of human beings.

The *"fish tape worm"* (Dibothriocephalus latus) is the largest of the tape worms, sometimes twenty-five to thirty feet in length. It occurs in European countries, Turkestan, Japan, Africa and other regions including parts of the United States. It is acquired by man by eating infected raw fish. Fish are infected indirectly by eating crustacea (water fleas) which have consumed larvae developing from eggs deposited in water with human faeces.

Symptoms of tape worm infestation are often lacking altogether. The patient may not suspect the presence of a worm until segments are discovered in the stools. Occasionally, there may be pain in the abdomen, capricious appetite and anemia, resembling pernicious anemia.

Diagnosis. By finding segments in faeces or on underwear, or ova under the microscope in stool specimens.

Prevention.

1. Thorough cooking of beef, pork and fish.
2. Proper disposal of all night soil. Faeces known to contain eggs or segment of tape worms should be burned.

Treatment. Whatever drug is used to rid a patient of tape worm, a period of preliminary fasting is essential to success. In particular no alcohol or fats are allowed for two days before treatment. After this, a dose of Epsom salts should be taken the evening before the medicine is to be administered. The next morning no breakfast is to be permitted before taking the drug. The treatment preferred by most physicians is a course of doses of aspidium, or malefern.

In case no doctor can be secured to treat the condition immediately after the diagnosis has been made, the lay person can try the old-fashioned remedy of pumpkin seed. Two or three ounces of the seeds are ground up and mixed with honey or syrup. All during the day before this mixture is to be given the patient fasts from solid food. On the evening of that day he takes a dose of Epsom salts. The next morning only coffee or tea is permitted before the pumpkin seeds are administered. A few hours after swallowing the seeds the patient takes another dose of Epsom salts.

In order to know whether treatment has been successful in expelling the whole worm, including the head, the patient should be instructed to pass all stools into a receptacle, mix them with water and strain them through coarse gauze. All segments thus isolated should be examined in the search for the head of the worm about the size of a pin head. This should preferably be identified under the microscope but its presence may be strongly suspected if the segments become smaller and smaller until the last one passed is very tiny. To prevent the worm from breaking before the head has been passed all effort to exert traction should be avoided. A very warm enema may be given however, to assist in the expulsion.

When it is not possible to be sure whether the head of the worm has been expelled it will be necessary to watch the stools for the possible reappearance of segments about six weeks later.

Cystocercosis. Occasionally the larval stage of the tape worm affects man. If, for instance, the eggs of the pork tape worm are swallowed by a human being his flesh may become affected similarly to that of the hog. The cystocerci, which are like tiny cysts, may cause him no inconvenience if they are located in the muscle tissue. If, on the other hand, they occur in the brain they may, after lying dormant for years, give rise to epilepsy.

Hydatid Disease

The echinococcus granulosis is a tape worm of dogs. Its larval stage however, may occur in human beings. Dogs become infected by eating the flesh of sheep harboring the larval form of the disease. Persons intimately associated with sheep-dogs or dogs allowed to eat slaughter house offal may ingest the eggs of the worm from the faeces of the dogs. As a result, cysts filled with clear fluid develop in the liver or other organs of the human being. This condition is known as hydatid disease.

Although the adult tape worm in the dog is only about one-eighth inch in length the cysts resulting from larval infection of human beings may become as large as a man's head. They often appear as tumors distending the abdomen. A skin test is available to assist in the diagnosis of cystic tumors from this cause.

Distribution. Adult tape worms of this sort may affect not only the dog but the wolf, jackal, fox, monkey and kangaroo. They are found in Iceland, Australia, Arabia, Algeria, Tunis, Egypt, Abyssinia, South Africa, Argentina and Uraguay as well as in Southern Europe. Wherever the worms exist in animals the cysts of hydatid disease may form in human beings intimately associated with the animals.

Prevention. Avoid contact with dogs in endemic regions and always wash the hands well before handling food.

Treatment. The only way to remove the cystic tumors of hydatid disease is by surgery.

Trichinosis (*Trichiniasis*)

The parasite Trichinella spiralis is a small white worm just visible to the naked eye. It is primarily a parasite of rats but pigs or wild boars become infected by eating diseased rats; and human beings contract the disease by eating undercooked pork. Pigs develop trichinosis also from eating garbage containing infected pork. The cooking of garbage before it is fed to swine removes this hazard.

When eating pork infected with trichinosis a person swallows hundreds of microscopic cysts. From these cysts adult worms develop in the intestine. The female worms give birth to myriads of larvae which travel by the lymphatics and veins and become encysted in the muscles. Here they may remain alive for many years but generally they die and become calcified after a year or two. In this disease the larval stage and the adult stage of the worm's development occur in the same host.

Distribution. Trichinosis may occur anywhere. It is not uncommon in the United States and is also found in Europe and in China and India. In Africa it is a menace to those who eat wild swine.

Symptoms. Many people who have never been conscious of symptoms are found at post-mortem examination to have signs of previous slight infection, especially in the muscles of their diaphragms. Severe infection, on the other hand, gives rise to violent symptoms. These may follow the eating of diseased pork after a period varying from a few hours to several days. Nausea, vomiting, abdominal pain and diarrhea are frequent symptoms. Those who develop diarrhea are fortunate since many of the worms are thereby washed out of the intestine. The taking of castor oil in treatment of diarrhea is a further aid in removing the worms. Sometimes no diarrhea or pain is experienced, but at a time from twenty-four hours to seven days after the pork has been eaten fever, sometimes accompanied by delirium, and swelling of the face occur. The eyelids may become so puffy that the eye appears to lie at the bottom of a pit, in the center of a mass of swollen tissues. After from ten days to three or four weeks the muscles of the body become tender and swollen. The whole body may be so painful that even the pressure of the bedding is almost unbearable. There may occur a transient rash similar to that of scarlet fever.

The active phase of trichinosis lasts about three to four weeks. After the larvae became encapsulated in the muscles acute symptoms subside. Muscular pains however may persist.

Mortality. The average mortality is 5 per cent.

Diagnosis. The fact that a patient is known to have eaten undercooked pork aids in diagnosis but sometimes no such history can be elicited. There is a skin test for the condition but this is not always reliable. Microscopic examination of the patient's blood in trichinosis reveals a characteristic excess of the blood cells called eosinophiles. This may be the means of diagnosis. Occasionally adult worms or embryos can be found in the stools. The presence of swelling of the face is very suggestive. As a last resort a bit of the patient's muscle tissue may be cut out and examined under the microscope.

Prevention. The thorough cooking of pork should be routine. One half hour of cooking should be allowed for every pound. Smoked meat and cured meat are not excepted.

Treatment. In rare instances the patient is aware of having eaten undercooked pork and can take a dose of Epsom salts immediately. Apart from this early measure, treatment must be symptomatic and supportive. Hot applications may give some relief to painful muscles. The diet should be very nourishing, including a good supply of protein and much fluid. The physician may prescribe the vitamin B-complex, calcium and iron in medicinal form.

Hookworm Disease (Ancylostomiasis and Necatoriasis)

Definition. Hookworm disease is an infection of the small intestine by either the Ancylostoma duodenale ("Old World hookworm") or the Necator americanus ("New World hookworm"). These worms look like a curved piece of thread about three-eighths to one-half inch long. They inhabit the small intestine of human beings and suck the blood giving rise to anemia.

Distribution. The hookworm, in one of its two forms exists wherever the temperature and humidity favor its development, being constantly found between the latitudes of 36° north and 35° south of the equator. The Old World hookworm is prevalent in southern Europe, Northern Africa, northern India and China and is also found in the Netherlands Indies, Burma, Malayan archipelago, the Philippines, South and Central Pacific islands, Portuguese West Africa, Japan, Australia and among the native Indians of Paraguay. The New World hookworm is the one usually found in southern India, Burma, Malaya, Netherlands Indies, the Philippines, Polynesia, Micronesia, Central and South Africa, the Southern United States, Central and South America and the West Indies.

Places where latrines are inefficient or absent and where the population goes barefoot are most likely to be centers of the hookworm disease. Persons such as farmers or miners who are constantly in contact with the soil are commonly affected. The poor suffer more than the well-to-do. In some rural districts 40 to 90 per cent of the population are infected.

Source of Infection. Eggs of the hookworm are passed in large numbers in the faeces. Within seven to ten days after stools are deposited on the ground larvae hatch out. These cannot attain maturity except in the intestine of a human being. The larvae usually pass through the skin of parts coming in contact with the soil, especially the feet. From the skin they are carried to the lung and eventually make their way to the bowel. They may, however, enter the mouth with food or with dirt on the hands and pass to the bowel directly. By the end of six to eight weeks after the larvae's entrance, eggs of the adult worm begin to appear in the stools. As many as a thousand worms may live in the intestine for as long as twelve years, biting the lining of the bowel and consuming the blood. Ill effects of infestation are due to loss of blood and to toxins absorbed.

Symptoms. First, an eruption, called "ground itch" appears on the skin at the point of entrance of the larvae. Indigestion and abdominal pain may follow later; but the essential symptom is increasing anemia. Patients do not appear emaciated because of puffiness of the skin. They may have a low fever and they become tired, weak and apathetic. The appetite may be poor but on the contrary it is often ravenous. The attempt to satisfy the appetite may give rise to indigestion. Infected children are poorly developed for their age and often have "pot bellies."

Diagnosis. Discovery of the eggs of the worm in the stools is easier after hookworm medicine has been given than before. In old infections there may be no eggs in the stools and anemia may be the only indication of the disease. Blood examination may give a clue through the discovery of abnormal numbers of the blood cells called eosinophiles.

Prospects of Recovery. Untreated cases usually become chronic but in severe infections death may occur after a few months. Results of treatment are good even in severe cases.

Prevention.

1. Building latrines to prevent defaecation on the ground.
2. Using night soil as fertilizer only after it has been buried or stored in water-tight pits for two, or preferably three, months.
3. Providing shoes for those who work on infected ground.
4. Using gloves when handling damp, infected earth or vegetables grown therein.
5. Either abandoning infected ground or treating it to kill the parasites. The latter purpose can be achieved by burning thickly-scattered straw on the surface of the ground.

6. Protection of food and drink from infection; and the practice of always washing the hands before eating.

7. Periodic inspection of employees in places where infection is common and examination of the stools of those who appear anemic or have indigestion.

8. Education of workers in order to gain their cooperation in prevention and treatment. The cinema is sometimes used for this purpose.[1]

Treatment. A number of remedies are used with success. These include thymol, oil of chenopodium, and carbon tetrachloride. At present the best drugs for treatment are hexylresorcinal and tetrachloroethylene.

Hexylresorcinal is used according to the instruction given under the treatment of round-worms (on page 196). This is a safe drug and the best one for the treatment of children, debilitated patients and the pregnant. It has the advantage of killing other kinds of worms which may be present.

Tetrachloroethylene may be the drug of choice for *mass treatment,* because, although a light evening meal and a purge may precede its administration, *no preliminary treatment is absolutely necessary.* For mass treatment the following procedure is recommended by Brown.

Dissolve a dose of Epsom salts in half a glass of water. The adult dose, 2 cc. of tetrachloroethylene is added to this and the whole shaken up and swallowed at one time. Any of the drug adhering to the glass should be drunk with additional water.

It is well to refrain from eating fats or drinking alcohol just before or after taking the drug. The purge should take effect before food is eaten.

Various workers report the removal of 77 to 97 per cent of hookworms by a single treatment of this sort. Round-worms, however, often co-exist with the hookworms and they may be stimulated by this treatment. For this reason when round-worms are present it is well to precede treatment with tetrachloroethylene by a dose of hexylresorcinal.

Treatment of anemia is very important in hookworm dis-

[1] The Walt Disney film called *Hookworm* can be obtained from the Institute of Inter-American Affairs, Washington, D.C.

ease, since most of the symptoms result from loss of blood due to the hookworm's activity. When no drug for removing the worms is available large doses of iron together with a nutritious diet containing meat may restore the patient to relatively good health but will not keep him so. In severe infections such supportive measures should precede and accompany the administration of the worm medicine.

Strongyloidiasis

Another worm, even smaller than the hookworm, is the Strongyloides stercoralis. It may be found anywhere, but especially in Brazil, Cochin China and Africa. Its larvae, like those of the hookworm, pierce the skin to gain entrance to human beings.

Symptoms occur in two phases. In the first or intestinal phase, diarrhea is the symptom noticed. In the second phase the lung is affected and bloody sputum expectorated.

Treatment. Gentian violet in tablets with a resistant coating constitutes the usual treatment. It is recommended that 2 tablets, each containing ½ grain of gentian violet, be given 1 hour before meals, 3 times a day for 16 days. In obstinate cases a solution of gentian violet is sometimes introduced through a tube into the small intestine.

22

MISCELLANEOUS TROPICAL DISEASES

THE PRECEDING pages deal with parasites of the intestinal tract. Other sorts of worms invade the lymph vessels, the loose "connective" tissue in various parts of the body, the veins and the substance of organs such as the lungs and liver. Diseases produced in this way are now to be described.

FILARIASIS

Definition

This term applies to a group of diseases due to invasion of the lymphatic system or connective tissues by filariae, threadlike worms which produce living embryos in the human body. These diseases are all conveyed by biting insects.

Filariasis of the Bancroft Type

This disease is due to the Filaria bancrofti, a hairlike, transparent worm three or four inches in length. Worms of both sexes are found in lymph vessels and glands. The female gives rise to an unending stream of living embryos, or microfilariae which pass into the blood. Microfilariae exist in the blood of many people who have never shown any symptoms.

In some countries microfilariae can be found in blood near the surface of the body only at night. By midnight three hundred to six hundred can be counted in every drop of blood examined. By 8 or 9 A.M. all the organisms have disappeared. If the individual is made to sleep in the daytime for three days the process is reversed. There is no satisfactory explanation for this nocturnal periodicity.

In contrast to the periodic or classical form of filariasis bancrofti just described, there is a non-periodic type which appears to be restricted to the islands of the South Pacific area.

Mode of Infection. Various kinds of mosquitoes convey the periodic type of filariasis in different countries. In India, the West Indies and the Philippines the Culex fatigans mosquito is usually the responsible mosquito. In the non-periodic variety found in the Pacific islands the Aedes scutellaris, a mosquito peculiar to that part of the world usually transmit filariasis.

The mosquito when biting an infected person, takes into its stomach with blood a large number of microfilariae. These undergo changes in the mosquito and larval filariae are produced which enter the mosquito's proboscis. After this when a mosquito bites, the larvae wriggle out of the proboscis and enter the puncture in the victim's skin.

Distribution. The disease is widespread in the tropical and subtropical world but is especially common in India, South China, the West Indies and the Pacific Islands.

Symptoms. Filariae are not poisonous to the system and most cases of infection produce no symptoms. When disease symptoms occur they usually result from obstruction of the flow of lymph or to a developed sensitization. The following are some of the possible manifestations of the disease.

Enlargement of lymph glands is a common symptom in the Pacific, non-periodic form of the disease.

Cordlike swellings of the lymph vessels in the groin and red streaks and swelling in the legs and elsewhere result from an inflammatory process due to the filariae and are accompanied for several days by chills, fever, headache and vomiting. These red streaks or inflammation always spread centrifugally.

Filarial abscesses, seated deeply between the muscles, are said to be common in New Guinea. Abscesses also occur about infected lymph glands, as in the groin or arm pit. Dead filarial worms may be present in the abscess cavity.

Milky urine (chyluria), a rather rare condition due to rupture of distended lymph vessels into the bladder is associated with the *periodic* kind of filariasis.

Painful inflammation in the hip or knee is an occasional symptom.

Elephantiasis may result from repeated attacks of filariasis. It practically never occurs except in native people exposed over a period of many years. In this condition the blocking of lymph vessels by calcified filariae results in enormous enlargement of the parts normally drained by these vessels. Periodic attacks of secondary inflammation contribute to the result. In 95 per cent of cases elephantiasis affects the leg or the scrotum. Less frequently the arm, the breast or the external genitals of the female may be enlarged.

Elephantoid fever may accompany inflammation of the lymph vessels, elephantiasis or other manifestations of filariasis. It occurs at intervals of weeks, months or years. This fever begins with a chill and ends with sweating and may easily be mistaken for malaria.

Prevention. As in the case of malaria, anti-mosquito measures are essential. Local health officers should be consulted as to methods needed to exterminate mosquitoes since these differ in different localities. Wherever the disease is prevalent both the infected and uninfected should sleep under nets and "foreigner's" quarters should be two hundred yards or more distant from native quarters. Those capable of infecting mosquitoes are a danger to the community.

Treatment. Hetrazan is said to clear the blood stream of microfilariae. Apart from this, rest gives relief when lymph vessels are swollen and fever is present. Sulfa drugs are useful in some instances. In advanced cases enlarged parts of the body may be supported by bandages or removed by surgery.

Foreigners, infected with filariasis need not fear sterility, impotence nor elephantiasis. Worms do not multiply in their bodies. Attacks of fever and swelling of the lymph glands and vessels will decrease and finally disappear within a year or two.

Loa Loa Filariasis

Cause. Infection with the loa loa filaria, sometimes called the "eye worm," is conveyed by the bite of the mangrove fly (Chrysops). These flies bite from sunrise to 10 or 11 A.M. and from 4 P.M. till dark. They prefer the shade to the bright sunlight.

Distribution. This disease is found in West and Central Africa and particularly along the Congo River and its tributaries.

Symptoms. Adult worms circulate about the connective tissue and appear beneath the skin where it is loose and soft. They may be seen about the fingers, on various parts of the trunk and also under the surface of the eye where they cause conjunctivitis with irritation and fear of light.

Migrations of adult filariae cause pricking and creeping sensations. As an allergic reaction to the worm "Calabar swellings" occur at intervals, generally on the back of the hand or forearm but also on other parts of the body. These are painless swellings about the size of hens' eggs. They subside in a day or two.

Prevention is practiced by the use of a mosquito net with a fine mesh.

Treatment. No drug is known which destroys the parasite. When worms appear under the skin or in the eye they can be removed through a small incision. Injections are sometimes given to desensitize against the worm and prevent Calabar swellings. Cooling lotions may allay irritation.

Onchocerciasis (*Filariasis Due to the Onchocerca Volvulus*)

Cause. The buffalo gnat (simulium) becomes infected by biting persons with the microfilariae in their tissues and thereafter conveys the disease through its bite to other individuals.

Distribution. This disease is widespread in West and Central Africa and is found, more rarely, in Uganda. It also occurs in certain areas of Southern Mexico and Guatemala.

Symptoms. Hard nodules develop in different parts of the

body. These contain both adult worms and larvae. The tumors vary in size from a pea to a pigeon's egg. They are painful when small but painless when fully developed. Their number may vary from 1 to 6 although as many as 150 have been found in one person. In Africa, the most frequent sites of tumors are the ribs, hips, knees, elbows, and back. When near the hip joint tumors may cause limping; and when they are situated in the head or neck larvae may enter the eye, causing inflammation and impaired vision. In Guatemala and Mexico nodules are usually on the head, particularly in the scalp, and eye complications are common.

In the skin the presence of large numbers of larvae results in either a mottled, papery appearance, especially on dark skin and in the region of the shin; or a thickened condition resembling elephant skin may appear, usually on the thighs and abdomen. Such abnormal skin sometimes becomes infected through scratching. This filaria is one of the possible causes of the skin condition known as "craw craw."

Prevention. A mosquito net with a fine mesh protects from buffalo gnats.

Treatment. Whenever possible all nodules should be removed as soon as possible. This can be done under local anesthesia. By removal, eye complications may be prevented. When not removed they are a means of infecting buffalo gnats and thereby spreading the disease.

GUINEA WORM INFECTION (DRACONTIASIS)

Distribution

Guinea worms are found in the Nile Valley, West Africa, Nigeria, Uganda, Iran, Turkestan, Arabia and India. In parts of Deccan (India) nearly half of the population may be affected at certain seasons and on the West coast of Africa nearly every Negro has one or more such worms.

Cause

The adult female guinea worm, measuring two or three feet in length appears like a heavy, winding thread under the skin of an infected person. When the worm is ready to discharge the embryos with which it is packed it secretes some fluid which raises a blister under the skin. A burning sensation causes the part to be immersed in water whereupon the blister breaks and a small transparent tube, the uterus of the worm, protrudes, fills with milky fluid and bursts on contact with cold water, discharging embryos. These swim about when shed in fresh water and enter the bodies of cyclops (water fleas). Infected cyclops are swallowed by man along with drinking water and afterwards, in the stomach, the larvae emerge from the dead cyclops and find their way into the connective tissues. Development into an adult worm requires a year. After attaining maturity, female worms work their way to the parts most likely to come in contact with water, usually the feet and legs. In India, water carriers sometimes suffer from guinea worm on the part of the back which comes into contact with the water skin.

Prevention

Drinking water should be protected from pollution by persons suffering from guinea worm. Adding potash to wells or raising the temperature of the water by a portable steam generator kills the cyclops. Barbel fish which feed on cyclops are sometimes introduced into wells. Boiling the water used for drinking purposes removes the risk of infection.

Treatment

Douche the part affected in water at every opportunity. After about fifteen or twenty days of this treatment the embryos should all have been discharged. Now exert gentle traction and wind the part of the worm which emerges each day on a match stick. Be very careful not to break the worm or great irritation and pain may result. At the end of each treatment of this sort apply a dressing wet with a 1:1000 solution of bichloride of mercury over the stick on which the worm is wound. Daily treatment in this manner will finally result in the complete removal of the worm.

A physician may be able to facilitate removal of the worm by injections of phenothiazine into the tissues at some distance from the worm or by injecting a solution of bichloride of mercury directly into the worm itself.

SCHISTOSOMIASIS (BILHARZIASIS)

Definition

This term is used to denote a group of diseases due to invasion of the veins of certain organs by several varieties of schistosomes. These parasites are trematodes or flat worms, called "flukes" because of their fancied resemblance to fish.

Urinary Schistosomiasis (Due to Schistosoma Haematobium)

Distribution. In Egypt 50 per cent of the peasant population is said to be infected. The disease occurs also in North, Central, South and West Africa, Iraq, Palestine, Arabia, Cyprus, Portugal and some other places.

Mode of Infection. Eggs of the parasite are expelled in the urine of those who suffer from the disease. The eggs hatch on coming into contact with fresh water and the emerging embryos enter the bodies of fresh water snails. In the snail's body infective larvae (cercariae) develop. These escape from the snail and burrow through the skin of persons who come into contact with the water as in wading and bathing. Penetration of the skin gives rise to itching and redness. Having pierced the skin larvae enter the blood where they undergo further changes. Adult worms develop after about six weeks and live chiefly in the veins surrounding the bladder. Their eggs are discharged into the lining of the bladder and are afterwards released with blood into the urine by the process of ulceration.

Symptoms. About four weeks after exposure, fever and hives may occur. There may also be a cough at this time. Usually not until three to twelve months or more later do urinary symptoms appear. These consist of varying degrees of local discomfort and pain accompanied by the passage of blood at the end of voiding.

Untreated, the sufferer often continues to pass bloody urine for years. Spontaneous recovery is seldom complete. Eggs of the fluke sometimes become the nucleus of a stone in the bladder. Infection may travel upward to the kidney or may affect the genitals and be mistaken for venereal disease.

Diagnosis. The disease is usually recognized by finding the distinctive eggs of the fluke on microscopic examination of bloody material passed in the urine. In some cases it may be necessary to examine a specimen of mucus obtained from the lining of the bladder by cystoscopy.

Prevention. Popular education is essential. No evacuation of discharges should be allowed near fresh water. Children and adults should be warned neither to wade, bathe nor fish in infected water nor to drink it. Drinking water should be boiled if possible. Clear water may be heavily infected. Ordinary chlorinization cannot be depended upon to kill the organism. Infected water is safe for bathing when it has stood for forty-eight hours. If doubtful water must be used for bathing it should be treated with copper sulphate (in a final dilution of 1:200,000) or with lysol, cresol or other antiseptics. Reduction of the number of snails in ponds, streams and irrigation canals is attempted by means of clearing away vegetation, periodic drying of canals and the addition of copper sulphate or other disinfectants to the water.

Treatment of urinary schistosmasia usually consists of the injection of antimony compounds. Among these, potassium antimony tartrate (tartar emetic) or sodium antimony tartrate are injected into the vein or fuadin into muscle tissue.

Intestinal Schistosomiasis (Due to Schistosoma Mansoni)

Distribution. This variety of fluke infection occurs in Egypt, the East Coast of Africa and Central and South Africa, South America and the West Indies.

Mode of Infection. Infection with this fluke occurs as in urinary schistosomiasis.

Symptoms. Preliminary symptoms are more severe in this disease than in the urinary variety. They consist of hives, abdominal pain, loss of appetite, chills and coughing. In one or two months or more symptoms of dysentery may develop and eggs of the fluke can be found in the blood and mucus passed in stools. Thickening of the bowel can be felt, like tumors, in the abdomen. Ulceration sometimes occurs around the anus and buttocks. Later, enlargement of the spleen and liver may be marked.

The outlook for the patient, in mild cases, is good on condition that adequate treatment is given. Chronic cases with dropsy and enlargement of the spleen and liver are difficult to cure although they may live for years. Prospects for recovery are especially poor when ulceration and tumor formation have occurred. Some patients die of lung complications.

The prevention and treatment of intestinal schistosomiasis are similar to those described in connection with the urinary variety.

Schistosomiasis Japonica (Due to Schistosoma Japanicum)

Synonyms. Katayama disease, Oriental bilharziasis, Eastern schistosomiasis.

Distribution. This disease is found in the Far East, especially China, Japan, Formosa and the Philippines.

Symptoms. These are similar to those of intestinal schistosomiasis, but more severe. A greater proportion of patients ill with schistosomiasis japonica become emaciated and develop enlargement of the spleen and liver together with distension of the abdomen with fluid. This is the most serious form of schistosomiasis.

Prevention. Snails which convey this disease live in inaccessible places and are difficult to exterminate. Dogs and other animals are susceptible to infection and serve as reservoirs.

Sportsmen, when shooting snipe need to wear high boots lest they become infected while wading in rice fields.

Treatment. Similar to that of other diseases of this group. This is the most difficult type of schistosomiasis to eradicate. New drugs under experimental trial may prove better than any of the remedies available at present.

OTHER FLUKE DISEASES

VARIOUS OTHER trematodes may cause disease in man. Of these only two will be discussed. The one, Pargonimiasis, is a fluke of the lung. The other, Clonorchiasis, is a liver fluke.

Paragonimiasis (Due to the Lung Fluke)

Distribution. This disease occurs principally in China, India, Japan, Korea and the Philippines.

Cause. Lung flukes (Paragonimus westermani) are reddish brown, thick and fleshy oval organisms about 10 by 5 mm. in size (roughly, ⅖ by ⅕ inch). Eggs of the adult flukes in the human being escape in sputum and faeces and give rise to infection of fresh-water snails. In the snail forms of the organism develop which infect crabs and crayfish. Man is infected by eating raw or improperly cooked crabs, of which Koreans are very fond, with the raw juice of the crayfish which is taken as medicine for diarrhea. Infection through infected water is also possible. The flukes after having entered the human body attain adulthood and produce burrows and tunnels, usually in the substance of the lung. These give rise to spitting of blood. Other organs, including the liver and brain, may be affected.

Symptoms. There is usually a chronic cough in this disease, accompanied by bloody sputum. Diarrhea and abdominal pain may also occur.

Diagnosis is facilitated by discovery of the characteristic eggs of the fluke in sputum or faeces.

Prevention. Sputum and faeces of infected persons should be destroyed in order to prevent pollution of fresh water. People should be educated not to eat uncooked crabs or crayfish.

Treatment. No drug is known which destroys the parasite in the human being. Improvement of symptoms is said to follow injections of emetine and prontosil.

Clonorchiasis (Due to the Liver Fluke)

Distribution. This is a disease of the Far East, including India, Mauritius, Japan, Korea, Formosa and China. In some parts of China 50 to 67 per cent of the native population are infected.

Cause. The fluke responsible for this disease inhabits the bile ducts of man and some animals. Eggs of the worm, passed with discharges into fresh water, infect the snail. From the snail infection passes in turn to fresh water fish of the carp family. Man becomes diseased by eating raw, inadequately cooked or even dried, salted or pickled flesh of infected fish.

Symptoms. Enlargement of the liver is sometimes accompanied by diarrhea and jaundice. Later, dropsy appears together with a very severe anemia which may prove fatal after several years.

Prevention. All fresh water fish should be thoroughly cooked before consumption.

Treatment. This is unsatisfactory. Intravenous injections of tartar emetic, fuadin or gentian violet are sometimes used.

LEISHMANIASIS

ONE VARIETY of leishmaniasis, kala azar, has already been described on page 158. At this point two additional forms of leishmaniasis will be discussed. These are Oriental sore and espundia.

Oriental Sore (Cutaneous Leishmaniasis)

Synonyms. Tropical sore, Aleppo button, Delhi boil, Baghdad boil.

Description. This is a sore which begins like a pimple, crusts over and breaks down into an ulcer which lasts six months to a year or even longer unless specific treatment is given. The ulcer is followed by a depressed and often disfiguring scar. The sores may be single or multiple. One attack confers immunity.

Distribution. In Baghdad almost everyone has scars of sores, and these are often on the face. The disease occurs in other parts of Iraq and in Arabia, Iran, Sudan, Palestine, Transjordania, North Africa, Egypt, Syria, Caucasus, India, Transcaspia, Turkestan, South China, West Indies, Central and South America, Mexico, Southern Italy, Southern Greece, Sicily, Crete, Cyprus and other places. Usually kala azar and Oriental sore do not occur in the same locality; but in Central Asia the two diseases exist together and neither affection surely confers immunity from the other.

Cause. Tropical sores are due to the Leishmania tropica, probably transmitted in most cases by the bite of the sandfly.

Direct inoculation from man to man, however, is possible. The disease exists notably in dogs, but also in cats, brown bears and horses.

Prevention. General measures against sandflies are indicated as in prevention of kala azar. Dogs with sores should not be allowed in the vicinity of residences. Prophylactic inoculation produces sores after two or three months and these protect against further infection.

Treatment. Intravenous injections of antimony compounds such as tartar emetic or, better than the latter, neostibosan or neostam are efficacious in the case of multiple sores. Berberine sulphate is sometimes injected around and under the ulcer; but this treatment is painful. The local application of X-ray in a single full pastille dose usually produces a cure in ten days. Carbon dioxide snow is effective if applied locally for 5 to 30 seconds, depending on the size of the sore, and repeated every ten days until healing is apparent.

Espundia or American Leishmaniasis

Distribution. This form of leishmaniasis is found principally in South America, Central America and Mexico.

Cause. The causal organism, the Leishmania braziliensis, is probably conveyed by the bite of the sandfly.

Symptoms. The disease usually begins with a sore on the skin, often on the margins of the ears. After this, ulceration occurs on the nose, spreading to the lips, mouth and throat. Multiple sores may appear on the body.

Treatment. For generalized sores antimony preparations are injected; but these are not always wholly effective for lesions in the mouth. Atabrine hydrochloride is recommended for injection into the base of sores, using 5 cc., or 10 per cent solution. At the same time 1 tablet (0.1 gram) of atabrine is given by mouth, 3 times a day for 7 days.

LEPROSY (HANSEN'S DISEASE OR HANSENOSIS)

Distribution

At the present time leprosy occurs principally in the tropics and subtropics. It is found especially in India, Africa, China,

Malaya, the Pacific Islands, the West Indies and the northern part of South America but also in many other countries. Many patients in the United States are isolated and treated at the leprosarium in Carville, Louisiana. Many infected persons also are at large. Leprosy has largely died out in the northern states. Only in the southern part of the United States does the disease increase indigenously to some extent.

Cause

The disease is due to the Bacillus leprae which closely resembles the bacillus which causes tuberculosis. Conditions favoring spread of the disease are humidity of atmosphere and close and continuous contact with infected persons, especially those suffering from the nodular type of the disease in which discharges are present. Leprosy is probably not hereditary although it tends to run in families. Children removed from their mothers immediately after birth usually remain normal. The mode of infection is unknown but is probably through the nose or the skin. With ordinary precautions there is practically no danger to attendants who care for patients; but long and close association in families spreads the disease.

Early symptoms

As a rule no symptoms are noticed until after a period of two or three years following infection. In extreme cases the incubation period may be as short as a few weeks, however, or as long as forty years. Early symptoms are vague and indefinite. There may be fatigue and mental depression; or the first thing noticed may be changes in some part of the skin, such as thickening, change in color or loss of sensation. In some cases contracture or atrophy of some muscles of the hand or foot, with resulting deformity, may be an early symptom. In other cases, quite suddenly nodules appear on the skin. The formation of crusts in the nose may be followed by nasal obstruction. There may be fever; and neuritis or arthritis may be so severe that the patient cannot move his limbs.

Sometimes before the development of nodules a rash appears. This is usually symmetrical on both sides of the body.

Patches may be pink, brown, fawn color or lighter than the rest of the skin. They may disappear and return. Loss of hair in the affected parts is striking, especially in the region of the eyebrows and beard. Gradually the deposition of leprosy bacilli causes thickening either on the skin or in the nerves. Deposits on the skin give rise to the *nodular* type of leprosy. Deposits on the nerves, on the other hand characterize the *nerve type* of the disease. Most cases are not exclusively of either type but mixed, with either one or the other type of abnormality predominating.

Nodular Leprosy (*Lepromatous Type, Cutaneous Type, Malignant Type*)

The nodules in this type vary in size from that of a split pea to great plaques many inches in diameter. Their color may be that of the surrounding skin, dirty pink, yellow or dark brown. They are devoid of hair and sometimes lacking in sensation. The presence of many nodules on the face gives rise to the so-called "leonine appearance." New nodules may appear and the old ones soften in the center and be absorbed or ulcerate and discharge sticky pus. The nose may break down, its tip become depressed and a foul-smelling discharge may escape from the nostrils. The eyes sooner or later become attacked and destroyed. Some other disease such as tuberculosis or pneumonia usually puts an end to suffering before leprosy has run its full course.

Nerve Leprosy (*Neural Type; Benign Type*)

In this form of leprosy patches of either a reddish or whitish color appear on the skin. They may have a ringed appearance. In other instances blisters may form. The border of these patches may be sensitive but the center is anesthetic so that if the surface is pricked with a pin no sensation is felt. Later, other abnormalities of sensation occur such as neuralgic pains or feelings described as "pins and needles." There may be fever and glands may become enlarged. The ulnar ("funny bone") nerve and other nerves sometimes become thickened so that they can be felt beneath the skin. Muscles supplied by the diseased nerves atrophy causing distortion of the parts and loss of power. Sometimes the eyelids cannot be closed so that the eyes become hard and dry and sight is lost. The nose caves in, lips are paralyzed and saliva dribbles. Ulcers forming on the hands and feet may cause fingers and toes to drop off. In other cases finger bones are absorbed giving rise to shortening of fingers.

Diagnosis

In doubtful cases the loss of sensation may give the needed clue. The centers of patches are quite insensitive. In no other skin disease is this definite lack of sensation found. Another clue may be discovered by examining the lobes of the ears and the eyebrows for nodules and the hands for contraction with distortion of the third and fourth finger especially. In the laboratory the diagnosis can be made by examination of the nasal discharge and by other methods.

The prospect for the patient is better in nerve leprosy than in the nodular type. Cases may be arrested and live for years, but relapses are likely to occur. Nodular leprosy saps the strength and makes the patient a prey to tuberculosis, pneumonia or other diseases. "Galloping leprosy" may prove fatal within a year from the beginning of symptoms.

Prevention

Segregation and isolation of lepers is a very important measure, especially for cases of the nodular type. Those of the neural type having no discharges are not so dangerous to the community. But these cases should report for examination every few months.

Children of lepers should be separated from their parents at birth. With this precaution they have a good chance of remaining normal, but they need to be observed frequently for evidences of the disease. Hysterical dread of casual contact with lepers is unjustified. Nevertheless lepers should not be allowed to beg on the streets, to frequent fairs, to sell or handle food or to become servants or prostitutes.

Like tuberculous patients lepers may contaminate their sur-

roundings with their discharges and excretions. Even more
care is needed to prevent spread of infection through dishes
and other articles used by lepers than in the case of tuberculosis.

Treatment

Hygienic measures in themselves do much to improve the
leper's condition. Good food, frequent bathing, clean clothes,
fresh air, light and agreeable work and recreation, with the
avoidance of fatigue, are among the resources for treatment
in leper asylums. *Chalmoogra oil* and *hydnocarpus oil* have
long been the most valuable drugs in the treatment of leprosy.
A preparation called *Moogrol* is given by injection.

Sulfones are now the treatment of choice in leprosy. These
include the drugs Promine, Diasone, and Promizole which appear to kill the bacilli entering the blood stream, preventing
the spread of the disease to new areas.

Many lepers need treatment for other complicating diseases
including syphilis, malaria or hookworm. Given all available
benefits, Chesterman estimates that one-third to one-half the
lepers met with in the tropics will become free from active
disease. Moreover, the danger of their infecting other people
is greatly reduced by treatment. No individual who has been
infected with leprosy should be discharged from observation.
Examinations should take place at periods of six months. Relapses are likely to occur at times when the general health is
poor.

YAWS (FRAMBESIA)

Definition

Yaws is a chronic, contagious disease closely resembling
syphilis and recognized by characteristic skin eruptions.

Cause

Infection by a microscopic "corkscrew" organism called the
Treponema pertenue is conveyed from person to person by
direct contact or possibly by flies.

Distribution

The disease is widespread in Africa, Ceylon, the West Indies, South America, the Pacific Islands, the East Indies, Papua, the Malay States and China.

Symptoms

About two to eight weeks after infection takes place there may be fever and other general symptoms together with swelling of lymph glands.

The Primary Stage. Soon after the patient begins to feel ill a papule, like a pimple, appears on some part of the body. It may be situated on the lower part of the leg, thigh, buttock, knee, arm, breast, lip or in other locations but seldom on the genitals. This papule may be so insignificant as to escape notice but it usually persists from two to four months or even longer, becoming covered by a yellow scab. This is known as the "mother yaw."

The Secondary Stage. About three months after the primary sore occurs the patient complains of pains in the joints and bones. Children may suffer from diarrhea and bronchitis and look thin and anemic. At this time scaly patches appear on the skin and yellowish red papules, thought to resemble raspberries, break out on the body. They discharge a yellow material and become crusted. Itching accompanies the eruption. Usually sores heal in a few months but the soles of the feet and the palms of the hands may never heal properly. This latter condition is known as "crab yaws."

The Tertiary Stage. A variety of disease manifestations may follow an attack of yaws, years after the initial illness. Among these are chronic ulcers which may form where the bone lies near to the surface, as over the shins, the collar bone, the bones of the forearm or the fingers. Ulceration may destroy the nose and the palate.

Diagnosis

A painless, encrusted sore occurring in a community where yaws is common is almost certainly due to yaws. The rash of syphilis may simulate that of yaws but it is generally pinker and not yellow like the eruption of yaws and does not itch. The history of a sore on the genitals or the presence of ulceration on the lining membranes of the throat favors a diagnosis of syphilis rather than yaws. The two diseases cannot be distinguished from one another by blood examination or other laboratory tests.

Prevention

All sores and wounds should be covered with protective dressings. Systematic campaigns should be organized for the treatment of all cases. It is recommended that houses or huts which are notoriously infected should be destroyed by fire.

Treatment

The same drugs used in treatment of syphilis are effective for yaws. Penicillin is probably the drug of choice. There is an immediate and striking response to treatment by intravenous injection of neorsphenamine or mapharsen. During the stage of eruption lesions disappear in the course of a few days. In the early stages of the disease one dose frequently effects a cure. In order to prevent relapses however it is better to give two or three injections. In the later stages when the bones have become involved prolonged treatment is frequently needed. Intramuscular injections of bismuth compounds are useful in treatment of tertiary lesions but are less effective than the arsenic preparations.

APPENDIX A

Revised by Mary Katharine Russell

I. RECOMMENDED DAILY DIETARY ALLOWANCES [1]

Revised 1948

Food and Nutrition Board, National Research Council

	CALORIES a	PROTEIN gm	CALCIUM gm	VITAMIN A b I.U.	THIAMIN c mg	RIBO-FLAVIN c mg	ASCORBIC ACID mg
Man (154 lb., 70 kg.)							
Sedentary	2400	70	1.0	5000	1.2	1.8	75
Physically active	3000	70	1.0	5000	1.5	1.8	75
With heavy work	4500	70	1.0	5000	1.8	1.8	75
Woman (123 lb., 56 kg.)							
Sedentary	2000	60	1.0	5000	1.0	1.5	70
Moderately active	2400	60	1.0	5000	1.2	1.5	70
Very active	3000	60	1.0	5000	1.5	1.5	70
Pregnancy (latter half)	2400 d	85	1.5	6000	1.5	2.5	100
Lactation	3000	100	2.0	8000	1.5	3.0	150
Children up to 12 yrs.e							
Under 1 yr.f	110/2.2 lb. (1 kg.)	3.5/2.2 lb. (1 kg.)	1.0	1500	0.4	0.6	30
1–3 yrs. (27 lb., 12 kg.) ...	1200	40	1.0	2000	0.6	0.9	35
4–6 yrs. (42 lb., 19 kg.) ...	1600	50	1.0	2500	0.8	1.2	50
7–9 yrs. (58 lb., 26 kg.) ...	2000	60	1.0	3500	1.0	1.5	60
10–12 yrs. 78 lb., 35 kg.) ..	2500	70	1.2	4500	1.2	1.8	75

(Continued on next page)

	CALORIES a	PROTEIN gm	CALCIUM gm	VITAMIN A b I.U.	THIAMIN c mg	RIBO-FLAVIN c mg	ASCORBIC ACID mg
Children over 12 yrs.e							
Girls, 13–15 yrs. (108 lb., 49 kg.)	2600	80	1.3	5000	1.3	2.0	80
16–20 yrs. (122 lb., 55 kg.)	2400	75	1.0	5000	1.2	1.8	80
Boys, 13–15 yrs. (108 lb., 49 kg.)	3200	85	1.4	5000	1.5	2.0	90
16–20 yrs. (141 lb., 64 kg.)	3800	100	1.4	6000	1.7	2.5	100

a Calorie allowances must be adjusted up or down to meet specific needs. The calorie values in the table are therefore not applicable to all individuals but rather represent group averages. The proper calorie allowance is that which over an extended period will maintain body weight or rate of growth at the level most conducive to well-being.

b The allowance depends on the relative amounts of vitamin and carotene. The allowances of the table are based on the premise that approximately two-thirds of the vitamin A value of the average diet in this country is contributed by carotene and that carotene has half or less than half the value of vitamin A.

c For adults (except pregnant and lactating women) receiving diets supplying 2000 calories or less, such as reducing diets, the allowance of thiamin may be 1 mg. The fact that figures are given for different calorie levels for thiamin does not imply that we can estimate the requirement within 500 calories, but they are added merely for simplicity of calculation. In the present revision, riboflavin allowances are based on body weight rather than caloric levels. Other members of the B complex also are required, though no values can be given. Foods supplying adequate thiamin and riboflavin will tend to supply sufficient of the remaining B vitamins.

d During the latter part of pregnancy the calorie allowance should increase to approximately 20 per cent above the preceding level. The value of 2400 calories represents the allowance for pregnant, sedentary women.

e Allowances for children are based on the needs for the middle year in each group (as 2, 5, 8, etc.) and for moderate activity and for average weight at the middle year of each age group.

f Needs for infants increase from month to month with size and activity. The amounts given are for approximately 6 to 8 months. The dietary requirements for some of the nutrients such as protein and calcium are less if derived largely from human milk.

1 Objectives toward which to aim in planning practical dietaries: The recommended allowances can be attained with a variety of common foods which will also provide other minerals and vitamins for which requirements are less well known.

II. RECOMMENDED DAILY DIETARY ALLOWANCES

(Expressed in Percentages of the Recommended Allowances for the Physically Active Adult Man)

	PROTEIN	CALCIUM	VITAMIN A [b]	THIAMINE [c]	RIBO-FLAVIN [c]	ASCORBIC ACID
Man (154 lb., 70 kg.)						
Sedentary	100	100	100	80	100	100
Physically active	100	100	100	100	100	100
With heavy work	100	100	100	120	100	100
Woman (123 lb., 56 kg.)						
Sedentary	86	100	100	67	83	93
Moderately active	86	100	100	80	83	93
Very active	86	100	100	100	83	93
Pregnancy, latter half	120	150	120	100	140	133
Lactation	143	200	160	100	167	200
Children up to 12 yrs.						
Under 1 yr.[f]	5/2.2 lb. 1 kg.	100	30	27	33	40
1–3 yrs. (27 lb., 12 kg.) ...	57	100	40	40	50	47
4–6 yrs. (42 lb., 19 kg.) ...	71	100	50	53	67	67
7–9 yrs. (58 lb., 26 kg.) ...	86	100	70	67	83	80
10–12 yrs. (78 lb., 35 kg.) .	100	120	90	80	100	100
Children over 12 yrs.[e]						
Girls, 13–15 yrs. (108 lb., 49 kg.) ...	114	130	100	87	111	107
16–20 yrs. (122 lb., 55 kg.) ...	107	100	100	80	100	107
Boys, 13–15 yrs. (108 lb., 49 kg.) ...	120	140	100	100	111	120
16–20 yrs. (141 lb., 64 kg.) ...	143	140	120	113	140	133

For footnotes see table I.

In Tables II and III, nutritive values for protein, minerals, and vitamins are expressed in percentages of the Recommended Daily Allowances for the average physically active adult man. Thus, you need not deal in different units of measure (grams, milligrams, or international units) for the different nutrients: all have been expressed in the same unit, a percentage, and for one type of person, the adult male (physically active), the amount of the recommended allowance is the same for each nutrient, i.e., 100. This makes it easier for you to evaluate any certain food. For example: for orange, the absolute values are 190 (International Units) for vitamin A and only 49 (milligrams) for ascorbic acid, but when stated in percentages of recommended allowance, the values are 3 and 65, respectively, and you know that orange is an excellent source of ascorbic acid and has only a little vitamin A. (Percentages may be converted to absolute values by referring to Table I for the value of 100 per cent.) Then think how much 100 grams represents in terms of a serving. For many foods it is an average serving. For example, 100 grams of bacon is 2 slices. But 100 grams of milk is only ⅜ cup, and 100 grams of cottage cheese is almost 1½ cups.

III. NUTRITIVE VALUES OF 100-GRAM (3½-OZ.) EDIBLE PORTION OF SOME FOODS²

(Nutrients expressed as percentages of the Recommended Daily Allowance for the physically active adult man.)

Food	FOOD ENERGY Calories	PERCENTAGE OF THE AMOUNT RECOMMENDED FOR A PHYSICALLY ACTIVE MAN PER DAY					
		Protein	Calcium	Vitamin A	Thiamin	Riboflavin	Ascorbic Acid
1. VEGETABLES							
Alibangbang leaves	36	1	3		6	9	15
Amaranth (Tampala)	21	6	27	120	9	9	100
Asparagus	21	3	3	21	9	1	45
Balsam pear (Bitter gourd)	29	1	3	3	6		70
Bamboo shoots	27	3	1	Tr.	9	3	6
Bean sprouts, Mung	23	3	3	Tr.	3	6	18
Beans, broad, incl. horse bean	98	12	3	3	18	9	40
Beans, green, snap	35	3	6	12	6	6	24
Beet greens	27	3	12 ᵃ	140	6	9	45
Beets, peeled root	42	3	3	Tr.	1	3	12
Betel leaves	36	3	15 ᵇ	180 ᶜ			6

(Continued on pages 230–239)

² Values are for foods fresh and raw unless otherwise specified. The classification is not botanical, but according to common usage. For other foods, or for scientific names, refer to "Tables of Nutritive Values" in "Suggested Reading" at end of chapter 10.

Tr. = Trace. Blank spaces indicate that data were not available or insufficient for imputing a value. For footnotes ᵃ to ʲ see end of table III.

PERCENTAGE OF THE AMOUNT RECOMMENDED FOR A PHYSICALLY ACTIVE MAN PER DAY

Food	FOOD ENERGY Calories	Protein	Calcium	Vitamin A	Thiamin	Riboflavin	Ascorbic Acid
Broccoli	29	6	12	70	6	12	160
Brussels sprouts	47	6	3	9	6	9	120
Cabbage, Chinese	14	3	15	55	3	9	60
Cabbage, common	24	1	6	1	3	3	65
Carrots	42	1	3	240	3	3	6
Cassava leaves	58	6	3	220	18	24	420
Cauliflower	25	3	3	1	6	6	90
Celery, bleached unbleached	18	1	6	0	3	1	9
Chard, Swiss, leaves and stalks	20	1	6	3	3	3	15
Chrysanthemum	21	1	9[a]	55	1	3	50
Collards	17	3	6	1	3	3	27
Coriander leaves	40	6	24	140	6	15	140
Corn, sweet	36	3	18	120	6	6	120
Cucumber	92	6	1	9[d]	9	6	15
Dandelion greens	12	1	1	0[e]	1	1	9
Drumsticks	44	3	18	280	12	9	45
Eggplant	32	3	3	9	3	3	45
Garlic	24	1	1	1			6
Kale	95	6	3	Tr.	3	3	18
Kohlrabi	40	6	21	160	15	15	160
Leeks	30	3	6	Tr.	6	6	80
Lettuce, headed	45	3	6	1	3	3	21
all other	15	1	3	12	3	3	9
Lotus root	15	1	6	30	3	3	24
	49	3	3		3	3	30

Mushroom, common	16	3	1	0	6	24	6
Mustard greens	22	3	3	120	6	12	140
Okra (ladies' finger)	32	3	9	15	6	3	40
Onion, mature	45	1	3	1	1	1	12
Parsnip	78	3	6	0	6	6	24
Peas, green	98	9	3	15	21	9	35
Pepper, green	25	1	1	12	3	3	160
Potato	83	3	1	Tr.	6	1	21
Purslane, leaves and stems	21	3	9	50	1	6	35
Radish, Chinese (Daikon)	19	1	3	Tr.	1	1	40
Seguidillas (winged bean, Goa bean)	33	3	6	15	15		9
Shepherd's purse	39	6	30	180			70
Spinach	20	3	9 a	6	6	12	80
Squash, summer	16	1	1	100	3	6	21
Squash, winter	38	3	1	160 f	3	6	9
Sweet potato	123	3	3	1	6	3	30
Talinum	30	1	12		12	9	70
Taro, leaves and stems	40	3	9	21	3	1	40
Tomato	20	1	1	Tr.	3	3	30
Turnip, white	32	1	3	200	3	24	35
Turnip greens	30	3	27		6		180
Water chestnut	54	1	Tr.				
Water cress	18	3	18	90	6	9	100
2. FRUITS							
Apple	58	Tr.	1	1	3	1	6
Apricot, fresh	51	1	1	55	1	3	9
dried, sulfured	262	6	9	140	1	9	15
Avacado	245	3	1	6	3	6	21
Banana	88	1	1	9	3	3	12

Food	FOOD ENERGY Calories	Protein	Calcium	Vitamin A	Thiamin	Riboflavin	Ascorbic Acid
Blackberries	57	1	3	3	3	1	27
Bread fruit	102	3	3	1	6	1	40
Cantaloupe	20	1	1	70 g	3	1	45
Carambola	35	1	Tr.	24	3	1	45
Custard apple	101	3	3	Tr.	6	6	30
Dates, dried	284	3	6	1	6	6	0
Durian	144	3	1	1	15	12	30
Figs, fresh	79	1	6	1	3	3	3
dried	270	6	18	1	9	6	0
Gooseberry, Indian	94						800
Granadilla (Passion fruit)	94	3	1	Tr.	Tr.	6	21
Grapefruit	40	1	3	Tr.	3	1	55
Grapefruit juice, canned, unsweetened	38	1	1	Tr.	1	1	45
Grapes—as Concord, Delaware, Niagara, and Scuppernong	70	1	1	1	3	1	6
Guava	70	1	1	3	3	1	400
Jakfruit	98	1	3		1		9
Jujube, dried	287	6	9				18
Kumquat	65	1	6	12	6	6	45
Lemon	32	1	3	0	3	Tr.	65
Lime	37	1	3	0	3	Tr.	35
Loquat	48	1	1	12			Tr.
Lychee (Litchee), fresh	64	1	1				55
dried	277	6	3			3	55

Mango	66	1	1	120	3	3	55
Orange	45	1	3	3	6	1	65
Orange juice, fresh	44	1	1	3	6	1	65
Papaya (pawpaw)	39	1	1	35	1	3	70
Peach	46	1	1	18	1	1	9
Pear	63	1	1	Tr.	1		6
Persimmon	78	1	1	55	3	3	15
Pineapple	52	1	1	3	6	1	30
Pineapple juice, canned	49	Tr.	1	1	3	1	12
Plantain (baking banana)	119	1	1	Tr.-24 [h]	3	1	18
Plum	50	1	1	6	3		6
Pomegranate	63	1	Tr.	0	1	Tr.	12
Prunes, dried	268	3	6	40	6	9	3
Pummelo (pomelo, pumelo)	48	1	3	Tr.	3	1	55
Raisins, dried	268	3	9	1	9	3	Tr.
Rambutan	52	1	3	0	Tr.		65
Rhubarb	16	1	6 [a]	1	1		12
Rose apple (Malabar plum)	56	1	3	3	Tr.	1	30
Sapodilla (sapota, chicos)	89	1	3	1	Tr.	1	18
Soursop	65	1	1	Tr.	3	3	27
Strawberries	37	1	3	1	1	3	80
Tamarind	239	3	6	1	21	9	3
Tangerine	44	1	3	9	3	1	40
Watermelon	28	1	1	12	3	3	6

3. MILK AND MILK PRODUCTS

Buttermilk, cultured, made from skim milk	36	6	12	Tr.	3	9	1
Cheese, Cheddar or American	398	35	70	27	1	24	0
Cheese, cottage, from skim milk	95	27	9	Tr.	1	18	0
Cream, light, table or coffee	204	3	9	18	1	9	1

Food	FOOD ENERGY Calories	Protein	Calcium	Vitamin A	Thiamin	Riboflavin	Ascorbic Acid
Cream, heavy or whipping	330	3	9	30	1	6	1
Milk, buffalo and carabao	106	6	15	3	3		1
Milk, cow's, fresh whole	68	6	12	3	3	9	1
fresh skim	36	6	12	Tr.	3	9	1
evaporated (unsweetened)	138	9	24	9	3	21	1
condensed (sweetened)	320	12	27	9	3	21	1
dried, whole	492	35	95	27	21	80	6
dried, skim	362	50	130	1	24	100	9
malted, dry powder	407	21	30	21	21	30	0
Milk, goat's	67	6	12	3	3	6	1
Milk, human	68	1	3	6	1		6
4. MEATS							
Bacon	630	12	1	0	24	6	0
Beef, carcass or side, med. fat	240	27	1	0	6	9	0
Ham, smoked, lean	389	24	1	0	45	9	0
Heart, beef, lean	108	24	1	1	40	50	6
Kidney, beef	141	21	1	24	24	140	18
Lamb, carcass or side, med. fat	317	21	1	0	9	12	0
Liver, beef	136	27	1	880	18	180	40
calf	141	27	1	450	15	180	45
pork	134	27	1	280	27	160	30
sheep or lamb	136	30	1	1010	27	180	45
Pork, carcass or side, med. fat	457	18	1	0	40	9	0
Veal, carcass or side, med. fat	190	27	1	0	9	15	0

5. POULTRY							
Chicken, hens	302	27	1	0	6	9	0
Duck	326	24	1		6	12	0
Goose	354	24	1		6	12	0
Squab (pigeon)	279	27	1		6	12	0
6. FISH AND SHELLFISH							
Cod, fresh	74	24	1	0	3	6	3
Halibut	126	27	1	9	3	3	
Oysters	84	15	9	6	9	12	12
Salmon, fresh, Chinook or King	223	24		6	6	12	
red, canned, solids and liquid (incl. bones)	173	30	27[i]	6	3	9	
Sardines, canned, drained solids	214	35	40	3	1	9	
Shrimp, fresh	84	27	6	1	3	9	
canned, dry pack or drained solids of wet pack	127	40	12			1	
Tuna, canned, drained solids	198	40	1			6	
7. EGGS							
Eggs, hen's, whole	162	18	6	24	6	15	0
white	50	15	1	0	0	15	0
yolk	361	24	15	65	18	18	0
Eggs, duck's, raw	189	18	6	24	12	15	0
limed	201	21	6				
8. SOYBEAN AND SOYBEAN PRODUCTS							
Soybeans, dry, mature	331	50	24	3	70	18	Tr.
Soy flour, full fat	347	50	18	3	50	15	0
Soybean curd	71	9	10		3	3	0

Food	FOOD ENERGY Calories	PERCENTAGE OF THE AMOUNT RECOMMENDED FOR A PHYSICALLY ACTIVE MAN PER DAY					
		Protein	Calcium	Vitamin A	Thiamin	Riboflavin	Ascorbic Acid
Soybean milk, without added nutrients	33	6	3				0
Soybean sauce	46	9	12	0	6	1	0
9. OTHER LEGUMES, mature, dry							
Beans, lima (butter bean, curry bean, Madagascar bean)	333	30	6	0	30	9	3
Beans, mung (green gram)	339	35	9	1	45	12	3
Beans, navy (also pea bean, white marrow)	338	30	15	0	45	12	3
Beans, pinto and red Mexican	349	35	15	0	45	12	3
Lentils, whole, entire	337	35	6	1	35	12	6
split, without seed coat	339	35	3	1	35	12	6
Peas, entire seeds	339	35	6	6	50	15	3
10. SEEDS AND NUTS							
Almonds, unblanched	597	27	24	0	15	35	Tr.
Cashew, roasted or cooked	578	27	6		40	9	
Chestnut, dried	377	9	6		21	21	
Cocoanut, fresh	359	6	3	0	6	Tr.	3
Ginkgo seeds (maidenhair tree seeds)	349	18	1				
Lotus seeds, dried	351	24	15				
Peanut butter	576	35	6	0	9	6	0

236

Food							
Peanuts (ground nut, monkey nut) raw, kernels with skin	548	35	6		70	6	0
roasted, kernel without skin	559	40	6	0	15	6	3
Pecan	696	12	6	1	50	6	0
Sesame (beniseed, gingelly seed, simsim)	568	27	120		60	12	
Sunflower seeds	569	40	10			6	
Walnuts, English	654	21	9		30		
Watermelon seeds	488	45	6	1			3
11. CEREALS, GRAIN PRODUCTS, STARCHES, AND STARCHY ROOTS							
Barley, pearled, light, dry	349	12	1	0	9	3	0
Bread, white, unenriched	275	12	9	0	3	6	0
white, enriched	275	12	9	0	15	9	0
whole wheat	240	12	9	0	21	6	0
Buckwheat flour, dark	347	18	3	0	40	9	0
Cassava (manioc), meal and flour	360	3	9		3		
Cornmeal (maize) whole ground, unbolted	355	12	1	9 d	24	6	0
degermed, unenriched	363	12	1	6 d	9	3	0
Flour, wheat, whole	333	18	3	0	35	6	0
patent, unenriched	364	15	1	0	3	3	0
patent, enriched	364	15	1	0	30	15	0
Macaroni, and other Italian paste, unenriched	377	18	3	0	6		0
Millet, whole grain	334	15	3	0	35	3	0
Oatmeal or rolled oats	390	21	6	0	40	9	0
Potato (see vegetables)							

PERCENTAGE OF THE AMOUNT RECOMMENDED FOR A PHYSICALLY ACTIVE MAN PER DAY

Food	FOOD ENERGY Calories	Protein	Calcium	Vitamin A	Thiamin	Riboflavin	ASCORBIC Acid
Rice, brown	355	12	1	0	21	3	0
undermilled or home pounded	363	12	1	0	12	3	0
parboiled	364	9	Tr.	0	15	1	0
enriched	360	9	1	0	30	1	0
polished, highly milled	360	9	1	0	9	1	0
Sago	360	Tr.	1	0	0	0	0
Sorghum, whole	332	15	3	0	24	9	0
Starch, inc. corn, etc.	362	1	0	0	0	0	0
Sweet potato (see vegetables)							
Taro (dasheen, yautia, cocoyam, tannia, eddo), corms and tubers	98	3	3	Tr.	9	1	6
Wheat, white, whole grain	335	12	3	0	35	6	0
Wheat, shredded, plain	360	15	6	0	15	6	0
Wheat germ	361	35	9	0	140	45	0
Yam	101	3	1	Tr.	6	1	12
12. OILS AND FATS							
Butter	716	1	1	65	0	0	0
Fats, vegetable, cooking	884	0	0	0	0	0	0
Ghee (clarified butter), low moisture	870	0	Tr.	40	0	0	0
Lard	902	0	0	0	0	0	0
Oil, red palm, unrefined	884	0	0	260	0	0	0
Oils, salad and cooking, all kinds	884	0	0	0	0	0	0

13. SUGARS AND SYRUPS					
Molasses, blackstrap	213	60	9	9	0
Sugar, brown	370	9 *j*	0	0	0
granulated	385	0	0	0	0
Syrup, table blends, chiefly corn syrup	286	6	0	Tr.	0
14. MISCELLANEOUS					
Chillies, very hot, fresh	85	6	15	9	65
Turmeric, root, dry	341	6	12	0	0
Yeast, dried brewer's	273	55	646	303	0

a Calcium may not be available because of presence of oxalic acid.

b Chewed with lime. Amount and utilization of calcium ingested with 6 betel leaves similar to 10 oz. cow's milk.

c Nutrient values are provisional only, calculated from values for fresh leaves; allows for 90 per cent loss of vitamin A during drying.

d Vitamin A based on yellow corn; white corn contains only a trace.

e Based on pared cucumbers; unpared have vitamin A value of 6.

f If very pale varieties only are used, the vitamin A value would be very much lower.

g Vitamin A based on deeply colored varieties.

h Vitamin A values range from trace in white-fleshed plantains to value of 24 for deeper yellow-fleshed varieties.

i If bones are discarded, calcium content would be much lower. Bones equal about 2 per cent of total contents of can.

j Calcium is based on dark brown sugar; values would be lower for light brown.

IV. DESIRABLE WEIGHTS FOR MEN AND WOMEN [3]

Age 25 and Over

Men

HEIGHT (with shoes)		WEIGHT IN POUNDS (as ordinarily dressed)		
Feet	Inches	Small Frame	Medium Frame	Large Frame
5	2	116–125	124–133	131–142
5	3	119–128	127–136	133–144
5	4	122–132	130–140	137–149
5	5	126–136	134–144	141–153
5	6	129–139	137–147	145–157
5	7	133–143	141–151	149–162
5	8	136–147	145–156	153–166
5	9	140–151	149–160	157–170
5	10	144–155	153–164	161–175
5	11	148–159	157–168	165–180
6	0	152–164	161–173	169–185
6	1	157–169	166–178	174–190
6	2	163–175	171–184	179–196
6	3	168–180	176–189	184–202

Women

HEIGHT (with shoes)		WEIGHT IN POUNDS (as ordinarily dressed)		
Feet	Inches	Small Frame	Medium Frame	Large Frame
5	0	105–113	112–120	119–129
5	1	107–115	114–122	121–131
5	2	110–118	117–125	124–135
5	3	113–121	120–128	127–138
5	4	116–125	124–132	131–142
5	5	119–128	127–135	133–145
5	6	123–132	130–140	138–150
5	7	126–136	134–144	142–154
5	8	129–139	137–147	145–158
5	9	133–143	141–151	149–162
5	10	136–147	145–155	152–166
5	11	139–150	148–158	155–169
6	0	141–153	151–163	160–174

[3] Metropolitan Life Insurance Company (March 1951). Reprinted by permission.

V. PERCENTILES FOR WEIGHT AND HEIGHT OF AMERICAN CHILDREN [4]

Of one hundred children, 9 will be smaller than the tenth percentile; 9 will be larger than the ninetieth percentile; there will be 50 children on each side of the fiftieth percentile.

PERCENTILES, BOYS			AGE MEASUREMENT	PERCENTILES, GIRLS		
10.0	50.0	90.0		10.0	50.0	90.0
			Birth			
6.3	7.5	9.1	Weight, lb.	6.2	7.4	8.6
18.9	19.9	21.0	Length, in.	18.8	19.8	20.4
			3 mo.			
11.1	12.6	14.5	Weight, lb.	10.7	12.4	14.0
22.8	23.8	24.7	Height, in.	22.4	23.4	24.3
			6 mo.			
14.8	16.7	19.2	Weight, lb.	14.1	16.0	18.6
25.2	26.1	27.3	Height, in.	24.6	25.7	26.7
			1 yr.			
19.6	22.2	25.4	Weight, lb.	18.4	21.5	24.8
28.5	29.6	30.7	Height, in.	27.8	29.2	30.3
			2 yr.			
24.7	27.7	31.9	Weight, lb.	23.5	27.1	31.7
33.1	34.4	35.9	Height, in.	32.3	34.1	35.8
			3 yr.			
28.7	32.2	36.8	Weight, lb.	27.6	31.8	37.4
36.3	37.9	39.6	Height, in.	35.6	37.7	39.8
			4 yr.			
32.1	36.4	41.4	Weight, lb.	31.2	36.2	43.5
39.1	40.7	42.7	Height, in.	38.4	40.6	43.1
			5 yr.			
35.5	40.5	46.7	Weight, lb.	34.8	40.5	49.2
40.8	42.8	45.2	Height, in.	40.5	42.9	45.4

[4] From data of H. C. Stuart and H. V. Meredith, as abbreviated and modified by E. H. Watson and G. H. Lowrey. (From *Growth and Development of Children,* Watson and Lowrey, published by the Year Book Publishers, Inc., 1951.)

PERCENTILES, BOYS			AGE MEASUREMENT	PERCENTILES, GIRLS		
			6 yr.			
40.9	48.3	56.4	Weight, lb.	39.6	46.5	54.2
43.8	46.3	48.6	Height, in.	43.5	45.6	48.1
			7 yr.			
45.8	54.1	64.4	Weight, lb.	44.5	52.2	61.2
46.0	48.9	51.4	Height, in.	46.0	48.1	50.7
			8 yr.			
51.2	60.1	73.0	Weight, lb.	48.6	58.1	69.9
48.5	51.2	54.0	Height, in.	48.1	50.4	53.0
			9 yr.			
56.3	66.0	81.0	Weight, lb.	52.6	63.8	79.1
50.5	53.3	56.1	Height, in.	50.0	52.3	55.3
			10 yr.			
61.1	71.9	89.9	Weight, lb.	57.1	70.3	89.7
52.3	55.2	58.1	Height, in.	51.8	54.6	57.5
			12 yr.			
72.0	84.4	109.6	Weight, lb.	69.5	87.6	111.5
56.1	58.9	62.2	Height, in.	56.1	59.6	63.2
			14 yr.			
87.2	107.6	136.9	Weight, lb.	91.0	108.4	133.3
59.9	64.0	67.9	Height, in.	60.2	62.8	65.7
			16 yr.			
111.0	129.7	157.3	Weight, lb.	100.9	117.0	141.1
64.1	67.8	70.7	Height, in	61.5	63.9	66.5
			18 yr.			
120.0	139.0	169.0	Weight, lb.	103.5	119.9	144.5
65.5	68.7	71.8	Height, in.	61.5	64.0	66.7

VI. SUGGESTED FORMULAS FOR WELL BABIES WHEN A DOCTOR IS NOT AVAILABLE [5]

BABY'S WEIGHT	EVAPORATED MILK FORMULA	FRESH BOTTLED MILK FORMULA	NO. OF FEEDINGS AND AMOUNT
8 pounds	Evaporated milk ... 7 ounces Water .... 13 ounces Sugar^a .... 2½ tablespoonfuls	Whole milk .. 14 ounces Water .... 6 ounces Sugar^a .... 2½ tablespoonfuls	5 feedings, 4 ounces each
9 pounds	Evaporated milk ... 8 ounces Water .... 15½ ounces Sugar^a .... 2½ tablespoonfuls	Whole milk .. 15½ ounces Water .... 7 ounces Sugar^a .... 2½ tablespoonfuls	5 feedings, 4½ ounces each
10 pounds	Evaporated milk ... 8½ ounces Water .... 16½ ounces Sugar^a .... 3 tablespoonfuls	Whole milk .. 17 ounces Water .... 8 ounces Sugar^a .... 3 tablespoonfuls	5 feedings, 5 ounces each
12 pounds	Evaporated milk .. 10 ounces Water .... 20 ounces Sugar^a .... 3 tablespoonfuls	Whole milk .. 21 ounces Water .... 9 ounces Sugar^a .... 3 tablespoonfuls	5 feedings, 6 ounces each
14 pounds	Evaporated milk .. 12 ounces Water .... 16 ounces Sugar^a .... 3 tablespoonfuls	Whole milk .. 24 ounces Water .... 4 ounces Sugar^a .... 3 tablespoonfuls	4 feedings, 7 ounces each
16 pounds	Evaporated milk .. 13 ounces Water .... 19 ounces Sugar^a .... 1 tablespoonfuls	Whole milk .. 28 ounces Water .... 4 ounces Sugar^a .... 1 tablespoonfuls	4 feedings, 8 ounces each

^{a} Use either granulated table sugar or corn syrup.

[5] From "Baby Book," prepared by New York State Department of Health (Bureau of Maternal and Child Care).

VII. *SOYBEAN MILK*

1. *Fresh bean milk* (from Bureau of Human Nutrition and Home Economics, U.S. Department of Agriculture).

Wash the beans and soak overnight in enough water to cover. Remove skins and grind the beans very fine, using a food chopper. Put ground beans in a cheesecloth bag, into a bowl of lukewarm water, using 3 quarts to each pound of dried beans; work with the hands for 5 to 10 minutes; wring the bag of pulp until dry. Boil the milk over a low fire for 30 minutes, stirring frequently; add sugar and salt to taste. Keep in a cool place.

2. In China, the beans are soaked in 6 times their weight of water, then beans and water are put through a stone mill. The product is strained through a cotton bag; the milk comes through and the residue in the bag may be used for adult food. Boil milk for 30 minutes.

3. *Modification of bean milk for infant feeding* (from Bean Milk Station, Methodist Mission, Peking).

To 1000 cc. of bean milk add

Calcium lactate	3 grams (or equivalent in bone meal)
Table salt	1 gram
Starch	30 grams
Sugar	60 grams

The starch is cooked in the bean milk; the calcium lactate is added after the milk is cool.

4. *Roasted bean milk* (from Guy and Yeh, of Peking Union Medical College).

Remove extraneous material by hand, then roast the beans by stirring with a little sand in an iron pot for about 15 minutes, until they are a light brown color. Sift out sand. Grind the beans in a stone mill; sift through a fine copper wire sieve, regrinding and resifting the coarser residue three times. The part which will not go through the sieve (about ½ the total) is too coarse for the younger infants, and may be used for older children. Prepare milk as follows:

Fine roasted soybean meal	500 grams
Bean starch	100 grams
Sugar	200 grams
Salt	5 grams
Calcium lactate	15 grams
Water	5000 grams

Mix the starch to a fine paste with a small amount of water and add this slowly to the mixture of roasted soybean flour, sugar, and salt, stirring to avoid lumps. At the last, add the calcium lactate very slowly. Add the remaining water and keep the whole at boiling temperature for one hour, stirring constantly. Restore evaporated water, stir the hot fluid well, pour into hot sterile containers, and cover with sterile covers. Mix well before using and warm the amount required for a feeding. (The dry soybean meal and supplements may be mixed and kept for considerable periods, to be made up as needed.)

5. Feed soybean milk in about the same amounts as would be used of cow's milk. If more than a liter a day is given, frequent stools may result. Supplement with sources of Vitamins A and D and of ascorbic acid.

VIII. *PEANUT MILK* [6]

1. *Preparation of peanut meal.* Shell the raw peanuts and dry them in the sun for several days. If the milk is to be used for young babies (under 3 months of age), remove the skins first by pouring boiling water over the shelled peanuts, and allowing them to stand until the water cools, when the skins may be easily removed by hand.

Grind the peanuts in a food grinder or pound them in a mortar. Put into an oil press and remove as much oil as possible. Dry the resultant peanut cake, pound to a fine meal, and sift until it is very light.

[6] Compiled from the methods used by several members of the Cornell short course for missionaries.

2. *Preparation of peanut milk.*

Peanut meal	70 grams	Egg	1
Mashed banana	150 grams	Sterile water	1 quart
	Calcium carbonate 10 grams [7]		

Add the boiling water little by little to the peanut meal, rubbing well after each addition to make a fine paste. Boil five minutes. Remove from the stove and pour back and forth from one container to another until it is cool, to give the appearance of milk. Add the calcium carbonate, well-beaten egg, and mashed banana.

"Milk" sufficient for 24 hours may be prepared once a day if it is kept in a very cool place.

3. *Use of peanut milk.* For babies under 3 months of age, syrup or brown sugar is used in place of banana.

Treat the peanut milk as if it were cow's milk, and modify it to make the desired formula, except that if bananas are used, no additional sugar or starch is needed.

IX. *ASCORBIC ACID FOR INFANTS*

Some source of ascorbic acid is recommended for infants, beginning usually about two weeks after birth. This is most commonly orange or tomato juice. Cabbage water and plantain water have been used for this purpose also.

1. *Cabbage water* (from Peking Union Medical College Diet Lists).

Cabbage	150 grams
Cold water	150 milliliters (cc.)
Salt	¼ gram

Boil the water; add the chopped cabbage; cover; allow to boil for 5 minutes. Remove from fire; allow to stand, covered,

---

[7] This provides about 4 grams of calcium, or 1 gram per cup of peanut milk. If more than 1 cup of peanut milk per child can be provided regularly, the amount of calcium supplement might be reduced correspondingly.

for 30 minutes. Drain the cabbage water from the leaves (discarding leaves); add salt to cabbage water.

2. *Plantain water* (from Methodist Congo Mission, Wembo Nyoma).

Cook well-ripened plantains in enough water to cover, until the fruit is tender. Strain off the water and give between milk feedings, beginning with small amounts and increasing until as much as 6 ounces is given daily.

I. INFORMATION ABOUT COMMUNICABLE DISEASES [1]

DISEASE	SOURCE OF INFECTION	TIME FROM EXPOSURE TO FIRST SIGN	EARLY SIGNS	PERIOD DISEASE REMAINS COMMUNICABLE	COMMON COMPLICATIONS	PREVENTIVE MEASURES
Chickenpox	Presumably infectious agent is present in the sores of skin, and in respiratory tract.	2 to 3 weeks.	Usually slight fever at the time of appearance of eruptions, which look like small water blisters; found on all parts of the body.	From the onset of the disease to about 6 days after the first eruptions, not more than 10 days.	Skin eruptions may become infected with other germs.	No immunization available. Avoid exposure. Almost everyone takes the disease after exposure.
Diphtheria	In discharges from the nose, throat, and any other mucous membranes containing the germs.	Usually 2 to 5 days. Sometimes longer.	Acute inflammation, especially of the tonsils, throat, and nose, accompanied by patches of grayish white membrane.	Variable; until germs of the disease have disappeared. Usually 2 weeks or less.	Paralysis of heart and throat muscles.	Immunization available. All children should be immunized against diphtheria at 9 months of age. The Schick test should be given 6 months later to determine whether treatment has been effective. If not, inoculation should be repeated.
German measles	Secretions of the mouth and throat, and possibly of the nose.	14 to 21 days.	Slight signs of a cold for 1 to 2 days followed by a red rash on face and body.	From the first signs of the disease for at least 4 days, and usually not more than 7 days.	None, usually.	No immunization available. Highly communicable. Most children take the disease during epidemics.

[1] From Lona L. Trott, *Red Cross Home Nursing* (The American National Red Cross, Washington, D.C.), pp. 403–408.

Disease	How spread	Incubation period	Symptoms	Period communicable	Complications	Prevention
Infantile paralysis	Nose and throat discharges of infected person and carriers, or articles recently soiled by them. Bowel discharges also contain the germs.	7 to 14 days.	Moderate fever, usually digestive upset, headache, vomiting, constipation, drowsiness, irritation, and stiffness of neck and spine. Later: paralysis.	Not definitely known. Apparently a few days before onset of disease and the first week or two of the disease.	Paralysis of affected parts of the body.	No immunization. Protection of children against unnecessary contact with people outside the home during epidemics. Isolation of all children with fever until diagnosis is made.
Influenza	Probably discharges from nose and mouth of infected persons and articles freshly soiled by such discharges.	Short, usually 24 to 72 hours.	Sudden onset. Fever 1 to 7 days. Excessive weakness, aches and pains in back and limbs, running nose, and sore throat.	Not known; possibly during the early, the acute, and the convalescent stages of the disease.	Pneumonia. Pus in the chest. Extreme weakness persisting for weeks. Meningitis. Heart disease.	Ask a doctor about immunization. Avoid contact. Patient should be isolated during the acute stage of the disease to avoid spreading it to others.
Measles	Mouth and nose discharges.	About 10 days, may be as long as 21 days when convalescent serum has been given, as a preventive measure.	Fever, signs of a cold in eyes, nose, and throat and early eruption in the mouth. Red rash and later scaling of skin.	From at least 4 days before rash appears to 5 days after the rash appears.	Pneumonia, chronic inflammation of the eyes, ears, and air passages.	Immunization of infants and children under 3 years of age with blood serum or whole blood of adults or older children who have had measles. Avoid contact with cases.
Mumps	Secretions of the mouth and possibly of the nose.	12 to 26 days. Most common period is 18 days.	Fever, swelling, and tenderness of the glands in front of and below the ears.	Probably beginning at least 1 to 2 days before swelling occurs and until swelling is gone.	Inflammation of sex glands in older children and adults.	No immunization. Avoid exposure.

I. INFORMATION ABOUT COMMUNICABLE DISEASES (Cont.)

DISEASE	SOURCE OF INFECTION	TIME FROM EXPOSURE TO FIRST SIGN	EARLY SIGNS	PERIOD DISEASE REMAINS COMMUNICABLE	COMMON COMPLICATIONS	PREVENTIVE MEASURES
Pneumonia (Lobar)	Probably discharges from the mouth and nose of infected persons who have the disease; articles freshly soiled with his discharges; carriers.	Believed to be from 1 to 3 days.	Sudden onset with chill followed by fever, often pain in the chest, usually cough and difficult breathing.	Not known; thought to be until the discharges of the mouth and nose no longer carry the infectious agent.	Pleurisy. Pus in chest cavity. Heart disease.	No immunization. Avoid contact with cases; avoid prolonged exposure to severe weather.
Scarlet Fever or Scarletina	Discharges from the nose, throat, ears, wounds, or skin irritations of a sick or convalescent patient; articles soiled, or used by patient. Carriers may also spread the disease; contaminated milk or other foods.	1 to 5 days.	Sudden onset with nausea, vomiting, fever, and sore throat, red rash on 2nd or 3rd day after onset.	Not known; 2 weeks at least.	Inflammation of the middle ear. Damage to heart and kidneys. Rheumatic fever.	No immunization; pasteurization of milk; avoidance of contact with ill persons.
Septic Sore Throat	The human nose and throat passages, usually the tonsils. The udder of a cow infected by the milker is a common source of infection.	1 to 3 days.	Acute sore throat appearing in epidemic outbreaks. Onset is apt to be sudden with a chill, high temperature, headache, and vomiting.	In man, presumably as long as there are any signs of the disease. The carrier stage may follow convalescence and last for some time.	Infected and enlarged glands of the neck. Middle ear infection. Arthritis, Heart disease. Kidney disease.	No immunization. Avoid exposure. Isolation of others during acute stage of disease and convalescence, and particularly exclusion of patient from participation in the production or handling of milk or milk products. Articles soiled with discharges from the nose and throat of patient should be disinfected.

		Incubation period	Symptoms	Period of communicability	Complications	Prevention and control
Smallpox	Eruptions on the mucous membranes and skin of sick persons.	8 to 16 days. Often 21 days.	1 to 5 days of fever, chills, headache, and backache; then an eruption appears first on the face and other exposed parts and then on the body.	From the earliest signs to the disappearance of scabs and crusts, which may last from 10 to 40 days.	Infection of the skin eruptions.	Immunization by vaccination which gives protection from 5 to 20 years.
Trachoma	Secretions and discharges from the eyes and eyelids of infected persons.	Not known.	Chronic inflammation of the eye and eyelids with formation of granulation.	As long as there are lesions and discharges from such lesions.	Scar tissue, deformity of eyelids and involvement of the eye itself, sometimes leading to blindness.	No immunization. Exclusion of patient from school classes. Isolation of patient is not necessary if he is properly treated and instructed in precautions against spread of the secretions of the eye to others by common use of articles. Period of communicability apparently may be shortened by appropriate treatment.
Typhoid Fever	Bowel discharges and urine of infected individuals. Carriers.	3 to 38 days. Usually not more than 21 days.	Headache, weakness, and continued fever, general body disturbance, diarrhea.	From the appearance of symptoms, throughout the illness and relapses during convalescence; until repeated examinations of the discharges show continuous absence of typhoid germs.	Hemorrhage from break in the intestinal wall. Bronchitis and pneumonia.	Immunization available which protects for approximately 2 years. Members of the household where disease exists should be immunized if they have not already had typhoid. Protection and purification of the water supply; pasteurization of the milk supply. Sanitary disposal of human excreta.

I. INFORMATION ABOUT COMMUNICABLE DISEASES (Cont.)

DISEASE	SOURCE OF INFECTION	TIME FROM EXPOSURE TO FIRST SIGN	EARLY SIGNS	PERIOD DISEASE REMAINS COMMUNICABLE	COMMON COMPLICATIONS	PREVENTIVE MEASURES
Whooping Cough	Discharges from the throat of an infected person.	7 to 16 days.	An acute infection invading the trachea and bronchi accompanied by a typical cough, usually lasting from 1 to 2 months. Irritating cough at onset and whooping develops within 1 to 2 weeks.	Usually lasts from the onset of the disease for about 3 weeks.	Bronchitis. Bronchopneumonia.	Immunization available but still in the experimental stage. It is of particular importance to protect children under 3 years from the disease. Child with disease should be separated from other children, and excluded from school and public places for at least 3 weeks.
Common Cold	Discharges from mouth and nose of infected person.	Probably between 12 and 48 hours. Possibly as long as 72 hours.	An acute inflammation of the upper respiratory tract. Usually slight fever and chilly sensations on first day. Running nose and eyes; may have sore throat and cough.	Thought to be limited to the early stages of the disease. Probably no longer than a week.	Sore throat; bronchitis; pneumonia; infected ears; chronic sinus infection.	No immunization. Avoid contact with persons who have colds. Isolate infected individual and prevent spread of discharges.
Impetigo Contagiosa	Eruptions on the skin of the infected person.	Not known but usually within 5 days and often within 2 days.	A condition of the skin characterized by pustules and scabs or crusts, commonly on face and hands, but may appear on body.	As long as the pustules remain unhealed and scabs are present.	Secondary infection of the skin and spread to other parts of the body.	No immunization. Highly communicable. Avoid contact with infected cases. Separate patient from others to prevent spread. Keeping the skin clean and in good condition helps to avoid the disease.

Ringworm of Scalp, Body or Feet. (athletes' foot)	Eruptions on scalp or bodies of infected persons; the scales and hair shed by individuals and lodged in damp places; articles of clothing, toilet articles, bathtubs, showers, and swimming pools.	Not known.	Skin eruptions on the scalp, the body, the feet, or the groin, depending on which form of infection it is.	Until the eruptions are healed.	None, but very persistent and often long drawn out.	No immunization. Avoid contact with persons having the disease. Avoid walking in bare feet around swimming pools, shower baths in public places. Keep the skin clean and dry, particularly between the toes. Children are more apt to have ringworm of scalp, face, and body. Adults more apt to have ringworm of foot.
Scabies (itch)	Persons harboring the itch-mite on their skin in burrows, particularly between the fingers.	24 to 28 hours. Length of time it takes itch-mite to burrow under the skin, lay eggs, and start itching.	Itching sensation. Later, sometimes inflammation due to irritation and secondary infection.	Until the itch-mites and eggs are destroyed.	Secondary infection and inflammation in neglected cases.	No immunization. Highly communicable. Avoid contact with cases, and with body clothing and bedding, bathtubs or showers, or articles used by infested person. Keep skin clean and in good condition to prevent the mite from having an opportunity to penetrate the skin.

II. *TEMPERATURE ACCORDING TO CENTIGRADE AND FAHRENHEIT*

C. =	F.	
0°	= 32°	Freezing point of water.
37°	= 98.6°	Normal body temperature.
40°	= 104°	Considered a high degree of fever.
62.7°	= 145°	Pasteurizing temperature.
100°	= 212°	Boiling point.

To convert Centigrade to Fahrenheit degrees, multiply the centigrade reading by 9, divide by 5 and add 32.

To convert Fahrenheit to Centigrade degrees, subtract 32, multiply by 5 and divide by 9.

Equivalent Temperatures

C.°	F.°	C.°	F.°	C.°	F.°	C.°	F.°
36.0	96.80	37.4	99.32	38.8	101.84	40.2	104.36
36.1	96.98	37.5	99.50	38.9	102.02	40.3	104.54
36.2	97.16	37.6	99.68	39.0	102.20	40.4	104.72
36.3	97.34	37.7	99.86	39.1	102.38	40.5	104.90
36.4	97.52	37.8	100.04	39.2	102.56	40.6	105.08
36.5	97.70	37.9	100.22	39.3	102.74	40.7	105.44
36.6	97.88	38.0	100.40	39.4	102.92	40.8	105.80
36.7	98.06	38.1	100.58	39.5	103.10	40.9	106.16
36.8	98.24	38.2	100.76	39.6	103.28	41.0	106.52
36.9	98.42	38.3	100.94	39.7	103.46	41.1	106.88
37.0	98.60	38.4	101.12	39.8	103.64	41.2	107.24
37.1	98.78	38.5	101.30	39.9	103.82	41.3	107.60
37.2	98.96	38.6	101.48	40.0	104.00		
37.3	99.14	38.7	101.66	40.1	104.18		

APPENDIX C

I. *SUPPLIES FOR TIMES OF ILLNESS*

▬▬

(These are intended especially for places where such provisions cannot be secured locally.)

An extra supply of bed linen to allow for frequent changes

Tools for the sick room
3 tested clinical thermometers for use in the mouth.
2 tested clinical thermometers for use in the rectum.
4 medicine droppers.
1 rubber hot water bottle.[1]
1 metal hot-water bottle. (This will be useful after the rubber one deteriorates.)
1 rubber ice bag.
1 rubber fountain syringe (enema bag) with assorted nozzles. (Fountain syringe and hot water bottle can be secured in combination.)
1 soft rubber bulb for syringing ears or giving enemas to babies.
1 small-sized rubber catheter.
A four-ounce funnel which can be attached to the open end of the catheter for giving high enemas to babies.
2 bed pans.
A pair of scissors.
A pair of splinter forceps (tweezers).
Box of wooden tongue depressors (a spoon handle can be substituted).
Box of wooden applicators for making swabs (any clean stick or a long hair pin, straightened out, can be made to serve).

[1] A rubber hot water bottle should be dried inside and out, blown up and stoppered when not in use. An ice bag or enema bag can be stuffed lightly with tissue paper. Before being packed, rubber articles should be powdered with chalk or talcum powder and wrapped in tissue paper. A catheter should be powdered, wrapped in tissue paper, and kept in a small tin box of its own. When not in use, rubber appliances should be put away in a trunk or tin box with a well fitting lid in order to protect them from contact with damp atmosphere.

4 half-pound packages of sterile, absorbent cotton.
1 dozen sterile gauze compresses in envelopes (3" x 3").
1 dozen sterile gauze compresses in envelopes (4" x 4").
6 sterile gauze roller bandages (width 1 inch).
6 sterile gauze roller bandages (width 2 inches).
6 sterile gauze roller bandages (width 3 inches).
2 ace bandages No. 1, for sprained ankles, etc. (width 2½ or 3 inches).
Adhesive plaster 1 roll (3 inches in width). A large supply is not recommended since it loses its adhesiveness in a hot climate. The plaster can be torn into strips of the desired width at the time of use.
2 triangular bandages, made from a square yard of muslin. These will be useful for slings and for first aid bandages.

Invalid foods for the emergency shelf

Saltines or "cream crackers."
Vanilla wafers, arrowroot biscuits or other simple sweetened biscuits.
Beef extract or bouillon cubes.
Vegex, for making vitamin broth.
Canned fruit juices (where fresh oranges and other fruits are not available).
Canned peaches and pears.
Dried prunes and prune juice.
Gelatine, flavored or unflavored for desserts.
Junket tablets.
Corn starch.
Barley flour for making barley water or gruel.
Tapioca or sago.
Macaroni, vermicelli or spaghetti.
Rice.
Cream of wheat, semolina, or farina.
Pablum (or similar baby cereal).
Strained and chopped baby vegetables in cans (where these are not easily made locally).
Cocoa.
Malted milk.
Evaporated milk in cans, or Klim or Dryco (when the supply of fresh milk is limited).

Lactose (1 lb.). This is milk sugar, mentioned in the fluid diet on
   page 93.
Butter in cans, if not available locally.

Vitamins and other accessory foods
(The amounts given are suggested as emergency supply only)
Ascorbic acid (vitamin C), 100 25-mg. tablets.[2] In time of illness
   these tablets may be taken separately or added to fruit juice or
   jelly, in order to increase the nutritive value of a restricted diet.
Thiamin hydrochloride (vitamin B_1), 100 1-mgm. tablets. Two of
   these tablets supply more than the required daily allowance for
   times of health. They may be given in tablet form or crushed
   and added to soup or cereal.
Calcium lactate, 100 6-grain tablets. Useful when sufficient milk
   cannot be taken as a source of calcium.
Mixed vitamin pills or capsules, such as Trapadin, or others made
   by reliable firms; package of 100. To be used as an aid to convalescence or to supplement a diet inadequate in vitamins, as
   for those who are dieting for weight reduction. 1 pill daily is
   sufficient.
Halibut liver oil capsules, packages of 100. 1 to 2 daily for convalescence from severe colds. These may be used also for the
   needs of older children who are underweight and for expectant
   and nursing mothers. To supply vitamin D as well as vitamin A
   halibut oil is available fortified with viosterol.
Aqueous concentrates of vitamins A and D. (These will not become
   rancid in hot weather.) A few drops daily may be used for
   babies as a substitute for cod liver oil. Drisdol is such a concentrate of vitamin D and Drisdol with vitamin A is also available.
Iron, for anemia.
   Tablets of ferrous sulphate (or Feosol tablets). One or two
   tablets may be taken by adults after meals and at bedtime. Older
   children in proportion.
   Elixir of ferrous sulphate (or Elixir of Feosol), especially suit-

---

[2] The recommended daily allowances for ascorbic acid are: men, 75 mg.;
women, 70 mg.; women (pregnant), 100 mg.; women (nursing), 150 mg.; children
under 1 year, 30 mg.; 1–3 years, 35 mg.; 4–6 years, 50 mg.; 7–9 years, 60 mg.;
10–12 years, 75 mg.; girls 13–20 years, 80 mg.; boys 13–15 years, 90 mg.; boys
16–20 years, 100 mg.

able for small children who cannot swallow tablets. Adult dose 2 to 3 teaspoonfuls in water, three times a day. Children should take 1 to 2 teaspoonfuls in water three times daily *between meals.* For infants begin with 20 drops daily (given between feedings 5 drops at a time.) The amount is to be increased gradually until two teaspoonfuls are taken in the course of the day. Administer in water or mixed with fruit or vegetable juice, preferably through a tube.

Medications usually available in kitchen supplies

Bicarbonate of soda (baking soda), 12-ounce can.

> For treatment of burns.
> For insect bites.
> Internally, for discomfort in the stomach. Dose ½ teaspoonful in a little water.

Powdered Mustard, 1 pound.

> For a *mustard bath* or *pack* in treatment of convulsions in children. Such treatment is not recommended in the presence of high fever.[3]

> Directions for giving a mustard bath or pack: Add 1 tablespoonful of mustard to each gallon of warm water (100°–103° F. or 38°–39.5° C.). If no thermometer is available test the water with the elbow. It should be warmer than the elbow but not hot.

> For a mustard bath bathe the child in a tub of the mustard water until the skin is reddened. At the same time apply cold to the head. Afterward wrap the child in a light blanket.

> For a mustard pack, which is preferred by some doctors, place the child on a blanket and then wrap him in a bath towel wrung out of the mustard water prepared as above. Apply cold to the head. Remove the pack after 10–15 minutes.

> NOTE: For treatment of convulsions warm water may be used if desired without the addition of mustard.

> For mustard plasters. These may be applied to the chest and back for a cold in the chest or to the pit of the stomach to allay vomiting.

> Directions for making a mustard plaster: Cut a piece of muslin twice the size of the surface to be covered by the plaster.

---

[3] Whether or not the child in convulsions has a high temperature, an enema of soapy water may be given. For an infant ½ to 1 glass of soapy water may be injected, using a catheter and funnel.

Make sufficient mustard paste to cover half the muslin, using 1 part of mustard to 2, 3, or 4 parts of flour, the degree of dilution depending on the sensitivity of the skin. For example, to make a plaster for an infant's chest mix 1 teaspoonful of mustard powder with 4 teaspoonfuls of flour and stir to a paste with a little *cool* water.

Spread the paste on one half of the muslin to within ¾ inch of the edge. Then fold over the other half.

Warm the plaster before applying it. This can be done by carrying it to the patient between two plates which have been warmed for the purpose.

Leave the plaster in place until the underlying skin is deep pink as in sunburn. This may take only a minute or two in an infant or as much as 30 minutes in an adult with a thick skin. Never allow blistering to occur. If the skin seems very sensitive on removal of the plaster apply oil or vaseline.

Table salt (sodium chloride), 1 package.

For gargling or the irrigation of sore throats. 1 teaspoonful of salt to a pint of hot water (see chapter 13).

For hot, wet applications to inflammatory swellings. 3 heaping tablespoonfuls of salt to a pint of hot water (see chapter 15).

A very dilute solution, swallowed lukewarm, for inducing vomiting. Glass after glass may be needed.

Salt solution in the strength of 2 teaspoonfuls to a pint of water may be used as an enema. When a patient vomits all food or drink taken by mouth 8 ounces of this salt solution may be injected into the rectum to be retained.

Useful drugs for the medicine closet (to be kept locked and out of the reach of children)

Laxative tablets, such as Phenolax wafers containing 1 grain of phenolphthalein, pleasantly flavored and scored for division. These are suitable for *occasional use* by adults and children (in doses proportionate to age). They may be injurious if used continually.

Epsom salt (magnesium sulphate), 1-pound can.

As a purgative. Adult dose 1 to 2 tablespoonfuls in just enough water to dissolve the crystals. For the best effect take on an empty stomach and refrain from drinking water until after the bowels have moved.

(WARNING: Do not give this or any other laxative medicine in the presence of abdominal pain and tenderness which may be due to appendicitis or other inflammatory conditions in the abdomen.

Externally, as a local application, using a solution of six heaping tablespoons of the salts to a quart of water. (1) Used cold, this makes a good wet dressing for poison ivy, or similar irritations. (2) Used lukewarm (preferably), it may be applied in wet dressings for burns. (3) As a hot solution it is useful for soaking inflamed parts of the body or in preparation of wet compresses to aid in "ripening" abscesses or boils. In snake bite it is used for wet dressings to be wrapped about the limb between periods of suction.

Milk of magnesia, 8-ounce bottle in liquid form or 100 tablets. each equivalent to 1 teaspoonful.

As a laxative. In liquid form 10 to 20 drops may be mixed with a bottle feeding for a baby of 3 to 5 months. Adult dose 2 to 4 teaspoonfuls.

To relieve "sour stomach." Take in same dose as for laxative.

Mineral oil. This should not be used habitually since it robs the body of fat-soluble vitamins. In emergencies it may be used as a lubricant to the bowels for constipation. One teaspoonful may be given to a baby or 1 tablespoonful may be given to an adult.

Castor oil, two 8-ounce bottles. Dose for an adult, 1 to 2 tablespoonfuls. Dose for a small child, 1 teaspoonful.

For diarrhea, to remove offending food. After this action it has a constipating effect. *Never use castor oil in treatment of constipation.*

To drop into the eye when irritation occurs from foreign bodies. Mineral oil may be used for the same purpose.

Bismuth subnitrate (or subgallate). *Powder:* 8 ounces. For diarrhea which continues after the patient has been treated with castor oil and a liquid diet. Dose: $\frac{1}{4}$–$\frac{1}{2}$ teaspoonful for an adult, repeated every 4 hours for several days if necessary. Bismuth causes the faeces to become black.

Kaolin, 8 ounces. Useful for chronic diarrhea. Dose 1 to 2 heaping teaspoonfuls stirred into $\frac{1}{2}$ to 1 glass of water. Repeat at 4-hour intervals.

Paregoric (camphorated tincture of opium), 4 ounces. Adult dose for relief of pain, 1 teaspoonful.

Pain-relieving doses for children, according to age:

Age 1 month   1 drop   1 year   5–10 drops
    3 months   2 drops   5 years   30–40 drops

After 5 years increase the dose gradually until at the age of 12 the adult dose is given.

Cough-quieting doses: For an adult, 15 drops. Children in proportion.

Uses of paregoric

To relieve intestinal colic, after the cause of the pain has been removed by castor oil. (Not to be used for habitual colic in babies.)

To relieve suffering in children during the course of acute illness. One pain-relieving dose may enable a child to go to sleep.

To quiet an incessant cough. The dose may be repeated every 3 hours while needed but its use causes constipation.

Tablets containing aluminum hydroxide, such as Creamalin or Amphogel, used for cases of ulcer of the stomach or duodenum and also useful for undiagnosed discomfort occurring habitually about 2 hours after meals. Two tablets are to be chewed and swallowed with a glass of milk or water.

Syrup of ipecac (or wine of ipeca), 1 ounce bottle.

For croup in children. Dose: 5 drops for a baby of a year or under. Dose increases with age up to 10 drops, repeated in an hour if necessary (see chapter 13).

As a "loosening" cough medicine for use when the patient cannot expectorate freely. Dose for children as for croup. For adults, 15 drops may be tried. An overdose produces nausea. It may be necessary to repeat the dose several times at three-hour intervals, but when the secretion has been loosened this medication should be stopped.

To produce vomiting (as in the case of poisoning). Dose: for this purpose, for a child ½–2 teaspoonfuls; for an adult, 1–4 teaspoonfuls.

Tablets of codeine, 100 ½-grain tablets. *A narcotic, not to be used unnecessarily.*

For *incessant coughing.* Adult dose: 1 tablet every 4 hours. This should be discontinued as soon as the patient can rest without it.

For severe pain which cannot be relieved by aspirin, give 1 to 2 tablets and repeat after 2 hours if necessary. For children's doses, see page 97.

Tablets of phenobarbital, 100 ½-grain tablets. This is habit forming and should be used only in times of special need.

For insomnia. One tablet, repeated after 2 hours if necessary. Not to be used habitually.

For great excitement or nervousness. As above.

For delirium. 1½ grain repeated after 4 hours if necessary.

Aspirin, Bottle of 500 5-grain tablets. For headaches and other aches and pains and for sore throat. Dose, 5 to 10 grains, according to the severity of pain. After this 5 grains can be given every 4 hours until relief is obtained. If aspirin causes discomfort in the stomach each dose may be accompanied by ¼ teaspoonful of bicarbonate of soda.

Aromatic spirits of ammonia, 4-ounce bottle. For faintness or whenever a stimulant is needed. (Never give in the presence of severe bleeding.) Dose ½ to 1 teaspoonful in a little water.

Tincture of Zephiran, 4 ounces.

Tincture of iodine, 2 per cent. Four one-ounce bottles with glass rod attached to rubber stopper. For local application as an antiseptic for wounds.

Cresol, 1 gallon of 2½ per cent solution. LABEL POISON. *For disinfecting faeces and urine* from infectious patients. Add in amount equal to the discharges and let stand one hour before disposal.

Blue tablets of bichloride of mercury, bottle of 25 7⅓-grain tablets. LABEL POISON. *These are very poisonous and must be guarded carefully.*

To make a disinfectant for the hands. Dissolve one tablet in a quart of water (a 1:2000 solution).

For preparing wet dressings for infected surfaces, as in treating boils (1:2000 solution).

Potassium permanganate tablets, 100 5-grain tablets. Solutions must be freshly made. 1 tablet dissolved in a quart of water makes a 1:5000 solution. This may be used for many purposes, among them:

For application to bad spots of prickly heat or for soaking the feet in acutely inflamed cases of athlete's foot.

For washing away foul-smelling discharges. It is good for use in syringing ears having a foul discharge.

Ethyl alcohol, 1 quart of 70 per cent solution.

For disinfecting the skin, as in preparation for hypodermic injections.

For rubbing the back (dilute with an equal part of water).

Boric acid powder (boracic acid), 1 pound.

As an eye lotion, made by dissolving a teaspoonful in 4 ounces of boiled water.

In the same strength, applied in the form of cold compresses in treatment of irritated conditions of the skin.

Zinc sulphate eye drops (1 grain of zinc sulphate to the ounce of distilled water).

For conjunctivitis, especially "pink eye."

Argyrol, 1 ounce of 10 per cent solution. The solution must be fresh in order to be effective.

As eye drops for eye infection.

For swabbing the throat.

or

Lunargen capsules, 12 capsules. One capsule dissolved in a small bottle containing a teaspoonful of boiled water makes a *fresh solution* for use in place of argyrol.

Paredrine hydrobromide aqueous, 1 ounce. As nose drops, to shrink the mucous membrane and open the air passages. This may be used for adults or children.

Olive oil or cotton seed oil, 8 ounces.

To soothe irritated surfaces, such as the chafed skin of infants.

Warmed and dropped into the ear for earache.

As an enema, to soften impacted faeces. ½ cup of warm oil, retained for several hours or over-night, followed by soapsuds enema.

Oil of cloves, ½-ounce bottle. For toothache. Clean out the tooth cavity, insert a bit of cotton soaked in the oil and cover with dry cotton.

Borated talcum powder, containing 10 per cent boric acid. For prevention and treatment of skin irritation, as in prickly heat.

DDT powder, 10 per cent in talcum. For lice. Several 2-ounce shaker-top cans.

Insect Repellent, "6-2-2" mixture. Several 2-ounce bottles.

Calamine lotion, 8-ounce bottle. For allaying skin irritation, as in ivy poisoning. (This should not be used on moist or hairy areas.)

Vaseline, 1 bottle.

For lubricating enema nozzles or rectal thermometers.

As a remedy for croup. 1 teaspoonful, melted, taken by mouth.

Boric ointment, one tube. As a soothing ointment.

Zinc oxide ointment, one tube. As a soothing ointment.

A burn ointment, such as Butesin picrate ointment, or tannic acid jelly, such as Amertan (the latter, containing tannic acid, should not be used on very extensive burns). 1 or more large tubes.

Sulphur ointment, 1 tube. For acne or various parasitic skin diseases.

Ammoniated mercury ointment, 1 tube. For impetigo and various parasitic skin diseases.

Desenex ointment and Desenex powder, 1 tube of the ointment and one can of powder. For athlete's foot and other ringworm infections.

FOR REGIONS WHERE MALARIA IS COMMON

Tablets of Aralen (Winthrop-Stearns, Inc., New York), 0.25 gram (base 0.15 gram). This drug is also called Chloroquine. 100 or 1000 tablets. (A large supply is indicated when suppressive treatment will be needed.)

or

Tablets of Chlorguanide hydrochloride in the form of Guanatol (Eli Lilly) or Paludrine (Imperial Chemicals Industries), 0.1 gram or 0.025 gram (for children), 100 or 1000 tablets.

FOR REGIONS WHERE AMOEBIC DYSENTERY IS COMMON

Carbarsone capsules, 0.25 gram, 20 capsules; or Vioform tablets, 0.25 gram, 100 tablets.

FOR REGIONS WHERE BACILLARY DYSENTERY IS COMMON (and also for pneumonia, blood poisoning and other serious infections where medical aid may not be available)

Sulfadiazine tablets, 100 0.5-gram (7½-grain) tablets.

FOR PIONEERS IN PLACES WHERE NO PHYSICIAN MAY BE
AVAILABLE IN CASE OF SERIOUS EMERGENCIES

Hypodermic tablets of morphine sulphate, 20 tablets, ⅙ grain with Atropine sulphate, ¹⁄₁₅₀ grain. These can be used orally as well as by injection.

Doses for children. In some instances, as in the case of paregoric, children's doses are stated in this list. Doses of anti-malaria drugs and sulfadiazine for children are stated in the text. It is also stated in the text that morphine should not be given to children unless absolutely necessary, and then in small doses (see pages 97 and 98).

Young's Rule: The proportion of the adult dose to be given to a child is usually computed by *dividing the child's age by the age plus 12.* Example: To find the dose for a child of three years in using a liquid medicine for which the adult dose is 1 teaspoonful.

$$\frac{3}{3+12} = \frac{3}{15} = \frac{1}{5} \text{ of 1 teaspoonful (60 drops)} = 12 \text{ drops.}$$

Sometimes the medicine to be given is dry. To a limited extent large tablets, such as those of aspirin, can be broken into halves or quarters, using a knife or scissors blade. For fractions of powders, or tablets which can be reduced to powder use a table knife to arrange the powder in the form of a square or oblong plaque on a piece of paper. Then divide this plaque into the desired number of portions which are as nearly equal as possible.

If the amount of the adult dose is too small to be easily divided, it may be diluted with powdered sugar, mixing the ingredients as thoroughly as possible. Then the mixture can be apportioned as desired.

Better than this method, in the case of soluble medicines, is the expedient of dissolving the tablet or powder in a definite amount of water, measured in drops or teaspoonfuls. Afterward the solution can be divided into the desired number of equal parts.

II. *WEIGHTS AND MEASURES*

The metric system is understood throughout the world. At present, however, the apothecaries' system is very frequently used in the United States and Great Britain.

The following tables are supplied in order that doses given in this book may be understood and converted, if necessary, into those of the other system.

APOTHECARIES' SYSTEM

Weight

60 grains	equal	1 dram
8 drams	"	1 ounce
12 ounces	"	1 pound (troy).

Volume

60 minims	equal	1 fluid dram (usually called 1 dram)
8 fluid drams	"	1 fluid ounce (usually called 1 ounce)
16 fluid ounces	"	1 pint
2 pints	"	1 quart
4 quarts	"	1 gallon

METRIC SYSTEM

Weight

10 milligrams (abbreviation mg.) equals 1 centigram. NOTE: 1 milligram may be written 0.001 gm. and 1 centigram, 0.01 gm.[4]

10 centigrams	equal	1 decigram (0.10 gm.)
10 decigrams	"	1 gram (1.0 gm.)
1000 gm.	"	1 kilogram (1 kg. [kilo])

Volume

1000 cubic centimeters (cc.) equal   1 liter.
(NOTE: 1 cc. of water weighs 1 gm.)

COMPARISON OF APOTHECARIES' AND METRIC MEASURES

Weight

Approximate Equivalents

1	grain	0.06 gm.
15	grains	1.00 gm.
1	dram	4.00 gm.
1	ounce	30.00 gm.
1	pound (troy)	360.00 gm.
2.2	pounds (avoirdupois)	1 kilogram or 1000 gm.

Volume

Approximate Equivalents

1	minim	0.06 cc.
15	minims	1.00 cc.
1	fluid dram (or drachm)	4.00 cc.
1	fluid ounce	30.00 cc.
1	pint	480.00 cc.
38.8	fluid ounces	1000.00 cc. (1 liter)
1	quart	960.00 cc.

[4] The abbreviation for gram (gm.) should not be confused with grain (gr.) of the apothecaries' system.

HOW TO CALCULATE PERCENTAGES FOR DILUTION

In the metric system this is self-evident (e.g., 1 per cent of 100 cc. is 1 cc.; 5 per cent of 100 cc. is 5 cc.).

In the apothecaries' system a 1 per cent solution always contains 5 grains to the ounce. Thus, to make a 10 per cent solution of argyrol, 10 times 5 grains, or 50 grains, of argyrol are added to an ounce of distilled water.

HOUSEHOLD MEASUREMENTS

For the use of those who have no scales or measuring glasses.

Liquids

1 drop [5] may be considered, for practical purposes, about 1 minim or 0.06 cc.

1 teaspoon, filled to the brim, may be considered 1 fluid dram (60 drops), or 4 cc.; a heaping teaspoonful of dry material, 5 cc.

1 tablespoonful is about 4 fluid drams, or 15 cc.

1 teacup usually holds about 4 ounces. Kitchen measuring cups have a capacity of 8 ounces. Whenever possible the measuring cup should be used for measuring amounts rather than the teacup. In this book "one cup" means a measuring cup, or 8 ounces, or 240 cc.

1 glassful, meaning a glass of ordinary size used for drinking water, may be considered to be 8 ounces, or 240 cc.

Solids

1 dram of a powder equals, roughly, 1 level teaspoonful.

1 ounce " " " " " 8 " teaspoonfuls.

---

[5] In reality the size of drops varies according to viscosity, specific gravity and the temperature of the fluid.

APPENDIX D

I. *AREAS IN WHICH VARIOUS TROPICAL DISEASES ARE PREVALENT*

(Refer to section II of this appendix for supplemental information and sections III and IV for information regarding immunization and precautions.)

All maps courtesy of U.S. Army Medical Museum

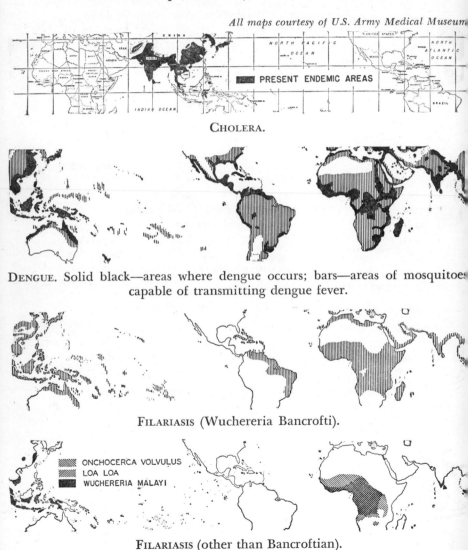

CHOLERA.

DENGUE. Solid black—areas where dengue occurs; bars—areas of mosquitoes capable of transmitting dengue fever.

FILARIASIS (Wuchereria Bancrofti).

FILARIASIS (other than Bancroftian).

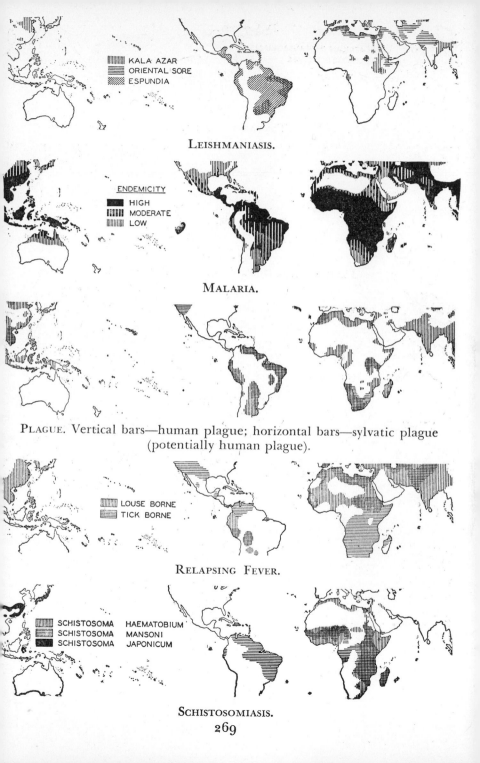

KALA AZAR
ORIENTAL SORE
ESPUNDIA

LEISHMANIASIS.

ENDEMICITY
HIGH
MODERATE
LOW

MALARIA.

PLAGUE. Vertical bars—human plague; horizontal bars—sylvatic plague (potentially human plague).

LOUSE BORNE
TICK BORNE

RELAPSING FEVER.

SCHISTOSOMA HAEMATOBIUM
SCHISTOSOMA MANSONI
SCHISTOSOMA JAPONICUM

SCHISTOSOMIASIS.
269

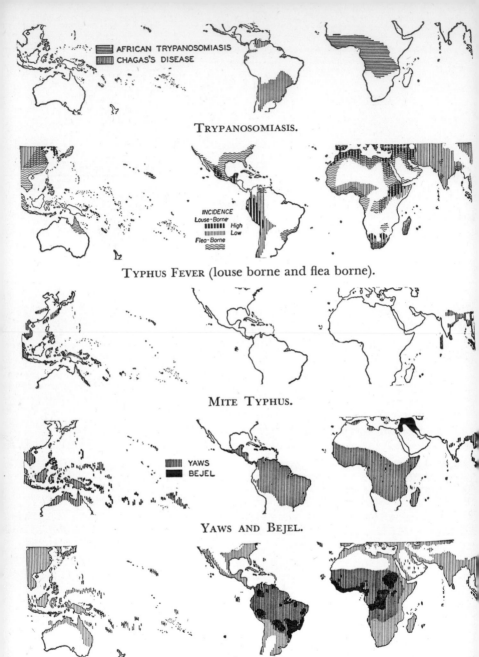

AFRICAN TRYPANOSOMIASIS
CHAGAS'S DISEASE

Trypanosomiasis.

INCIDENCE
Louse-Borne
High
Low
Flea-Borne

Typhus Fever (louse borne and flea borne).

Mite Typhus.

YAWS
BEJEL

Yaws and Bejel.

Yellow Fever. Solid black—areas of yellow fever; heavy bars—potential yellow fever areas; light bars—vector areas.

II. SOME DISEASES OCCURRING IN AFRICA, CENTRAL AND SOUTH AMERICA, AND ASIA [1]

AFRICA (Central, South, and the West Coast)

Note: For each of the diseases listed below and in the following lists, the general precautions of classes I and II (pages 276–278) are needed. In addition, extra precautions are needed for certain of the diseases. These are indicated by the numbers and letters following the names of the diseases. Such numbers refer to the class III list on pages 278–279.

A disease may be found in one part of an area and be absent from another part only a few miles distant.

Malaria (III, 9*a*)
The dysenteries: amoebic and bacillary (III, 9*b* and *c*)
Diarrheas of various kinds
Typhoid and paratyphoid fever (III, 8)
Dengue
Typhus fever, louse borne and flea borne [2] (III, 8)
Filariasis, including Bancroftian, loa loa, and onchocerciasis (III, 5)
Kala azar (leishmaniasis)
Myiasis (Congo floor maggot) (III, 6)
Oriental sore (leishmaniasis) (III, 3)
Plague (at time of epidemics) (III, 8)
Relapsing fever: tick borne (African tick fever). (Louse-borne variety also found.) (III, 9*d;* III, 7)
Schistosomiasis: Haematobium and Mansoni (III, 1)
Trypanosomiasis: African ("sleeping sickness")
Tick typhus: South African tick-bite fever; Boutonneuse fever (III, 7)
Yaws (III, 3)
Yellow fever (III, 8)

---

[1] Adapted from Department of the Army pamphlets Nos. 8-1, 8-2, 8-3, and 8-4 (Government Printing Office, Washington, D.C., 1943).
[2] The first six items are found in all tropical areas.

CENTRAL AND SOUTH AMERICA AND THE CARIBBEAN AREA

Malaria (III, 9a)
The dysenteries: amoebic and bacillary (III, 9b and c)
Diarrheas of various kinds
Typhoid and paratyphoid fever (III, 8)
Dengue
Typhus fever: louse borne and flea borne (III, 8)
Trypanosomiasis (Chagas' disease)
Echinococcosis (III, 4)
Espundia (leishmaniasis)
Filariasis: Bancroftian; onchocerciasis (in western Guatemala) (III, 5)
Myiasis (III, 6)
Plague (at time of epidemics) (III, 8)
Relapsing fever: tick borne (III, 7)
Schistosomiasis ("fluke disease"): Mansoni (III, 1)
Trichinosis
Undulant fever
Yaws (III, 3)
Yellow fever (III, 8)

SOUTHERN AND EASTERN MEDITERRANEAN SEA, RED SEA, AND PERSIAN GULF AREA

Malaria (III, 9a)
The dysenteries: amoebic and bacillary (III, 9b and c)
Diarrheas of various kinds
Typhoid and paratyphoid fever (III, 8)
Dengue
Typhus fever: louse-borne and flea-borne (III, 8)
Cholera (III, 8)
Dracontiasis
Echinococcosis (III, 4)
Filariasis: Bancroftian
Kala azar (leishmaniasis)
Oriental sore (leishmaniasis) (III, 3)
Plague (at time of epidemics) (III, 8)
Relapsing fever: tick borne and louse borne (III, 7)
Schistosomiasis: Mansoni and Haematobium (III, 1)

Trichinosis
Undulant fever
Yaws and bejel (III, 3)

THE FAR EAST

(Southern Asia, Eastern Asia, and the Netherlands East Indies)

Malaria (III, 9a)
The dysenteries: amoebic and bacillary (III, 9b and c)
Diarrheas of various kinds
Typhoid and paratyphoid fever (III, 8)
Dengue
Typhus fever: louse borne and flea borne (III, 8)
Chlonorciasis
Cholera (III, 8)
Filariasis: Bancroftian and Malay
Fish tape worm
Hookworm disease (ancylostomiasis) (III, 2)
Kala azar (leishmaniasis)
Oriental sore (leishmaniasis) (III, 3)
Paragonimiasis
Plague (at time of epidemics) (III, 8)
Relapsing fever: louse borne
Schistosomiasis: Japonicum (III, 1)
Trichinosis
Mite typhus
Yaws (III, 3)

III. *IMMUNIZATIONS* [3]

See sections I and II of this appendix for the areas in which tropical diseases are prevalent.

Due to constantly changing situations, there may be changes in the immunization program from time to time; hence this summary should not be considered to be an outline of permanent policy. Most travelers are informed at the time of obtaining a passport as to immunization and health certificate

[3] Adapted from Department of the Army pamphlets Nos. 8-1, 8-2, 8-3, and 8-4 (Government Printing Office, Washington, D.C., 1943). See also *Health Hints for the Tropics* (see bibliography, page 19).

requirements in their own specific instance. In any event, information can be secured from the Office of International Health Relations, Public Health Service, Washington, D.C. A booklet, *Immunization Information for International Travel*, and a supplement supplied with this booklet to bring it up to date can be secured from the Superintendent of Documents, Government Printing Office, Washington 25, D.C., at a cost of 20 cents.

All immunizations except that for yellow fever may be done by the traveler's personal physician.

Yellow fever inoculations are given by the U.S. Public Health Service in the following cities:

Baltimore, Md.	Miami, Fla. (inoculations also
Boston, Mass.	given at the airport)
Chamblee, Ga.	New Orleans, La.
Chicago, Ill.	New York, N.Y.
Cleveland, Ohio	Philadelphia, Pa.
Detroit, Mich.	Pittsburgh, Pa.
Fort Worth, Texas	Portland, Ore.
Galveston, Texas	San Francisco, Calif.
Honolulu, T.H.	San Juan, P.R.
Kirkwood, Mo.	Savannah, Ga.
Los Angeles, Calif.	Seattle, Wash.
Memphis, Tenn.	Washington, D.C.

Inoculations are also given at the following places:

Brownsville, Texas: U.S. Quarantine Station
Hamilton, Montana: Rocky Mountain Laboratory
Kansas City, Mo.: Director of Medical Services, Trans-World Airlines
Tampa, Fla.: U.S. Quarantine Station

The supplement to *Immunization Information for International Travel* keeps this list up to date.

An *International Certificate of Immunization,* usually supplied to the traveler by travel agencies, must be signed by the doctor responsible for each immunization. After this the signature of a government health officer must be affixed.

GENERAL INFORMATION ABOUT IMMUNIZATION [4]

	NO. DOSES (BASIC SERIES)	TIME REQUIRED (DAYS) (BASIC SERIES)
Routine immunizations.		
(1) Smallpox	1	. . .
(2) Typhoid-paratyphoid	3	14
(3) Tetanus	3	42
(4) Diphtheria	4	44
Special immunizations.		
(1) Yellow fever	1	. . .
(2) Cholera	2	7
(3) Typhus	2	14
(4) Plague	2	7

Routine Immunizations

Smallpox and typhoid-paratyphoid. Travelers must have been vaccinated against smallpox, typhoid, and the paratyphoid fevers within 12 months prior to departure.

Tetanus. Initial tetanus immunization (three doses). An additional dose (1 cc.) is required unless the routine initial immunization or a stimulating dose has been administered within 6 months prior to departure.

Special Immunizations

Yellow Fever. Yellow fever vaccination has been required for travelers to the following areas (see the solid black and heavy-barred areas on the yellow fever map on page 270):

Africa: between 16° N. and 12° S., including the islands adjacent.

South America: betweeen 13° N. and 30° S., including the islands, the Republic of Panama, and the Canal Zone. If travel is by air, this vaccination should be done at least 2 weeks before departure in order to avoid delays en route which otherwise might arise from the quarantine requirements of certain foreign governments. Documentary proof of such vaccination is required of persons traveling by air. Ceylon, India, and Pakistan require vaccination not less than 15 days prior to arrival for all persons.

[4] This must be checked for subsequent changes in requirements.

Cholera. Cholera vaccination has been required for travelers to Asia, including the Middle East and islands of the East Indies.

Typhus. Typhus vaccination has been required for travelers to Asia, Africa, Europe (including the British Isles), and the mountainous regions of Central and South America (including Mexico but excepting Panama).

Plague. Plague vaccine is to be administered only when travelers are under serious threat of exposure to epidemics of human plague.

Inquiry should be made as to the necessity of securing a *certificate of good physical and mental health,* signed by a physician, a requirement, in the past, of the following countries:

Morocco, French	Brazil
El Salvador	Chile
Nicaragua	Ecuador
Guam	Paraguay
In South America	Peru
Argentine	Uruguay
Bolivia	Venezuela

IV. *PRECAUTIONS AGAINST TROPICAL DISEASES*

CLASS I

FOOD AND DRINK PRECAUTIONS—ALL AREAS

Precautions against unsafe food

Permitted foods

Meat and fowl, well cooked and eaten hot. Or meat, fowl, or sea food straight from a can.[5]

Fresh vegetables and fruits, cooked and eaten hot.

Butter and cheese, straight from a can, or cooked and hot.

[5] The precautions "straight from a can" and "eaten hot" are designed to avoid contamination of food by unsafe containers or the hands of diseased food handlers.

Canned fruit or vegetables, straight from a can, or cooked
and hot. Oranges and bananas and other fruits with
thick skin, peeled by the consumer after pouring boiling water over it. Also tomatoes which have been
dipped in boiling water and are peeled by the consumer.

Bread or rolls, preferably straight from the oven. Cookies
or crackers from a can. Baked food can be made safe
by rebaking. Sweets of known make are safe, taken
from a can.

Foods not permitted

Sea food, doubtfully fresh or uncooked.

Meat which is not well cooked and hot or direct from a
can.

Locally made butter or cheese, unless cooked and hot.

Ice cream.

Custard-type foods, such as cream puffs and custards.

Salads and raw fruits (with the exceptions mentioned
above). Anything which has had contact with lettuce.
Cut-up fruits or canned fruit to which cream or custard
sauce has been added.

Foods which have been exposed to flies.

Foods which have had contact with ice.

Always wash your hands before eating.

Precautions against unsafe drinks

Drinks permitted

Water which has been boiled for 5 minutes and has not
been contaminated afterward.

Water to which tincture of iodine has been added, drop
by drop until a faint yellow tinge is seen, and has afterward been allowed to stand for 15 minutes.

Water to which disinfecting tablets of Globaline have
been added.

Imported water and other drinks in bottles with unbroken seals, opened at the table. Drinks bottled at the
hotel or restaurant, including imported bottles refilled,
are unsafe.

Milk and cream which have been boiled or pasteurized, or canned products, direct from the can and undiluted.

The milk of green coconuts, opened by the consumer.

Hot tea and coffee and other hot drinks, to which no unsafe milk or cream has been added.

Drinks not permitted

All drinks not conforming to the above requirements and those which have had contact with flies.

Drinks containing ice.

CLASS II

PRECAUTIONS AGAINST INSECT-BORNE DISEASES—ALL AREAS

The use of a bed net (may be purchased from government surplus stores or sporting goods stores).

The use of insecticide bombs.

The use of repellents.

Wearing of protective clothing, e.g., head nets, long sleeves, and high boots, at times of exposure to flying insects.

Refraining from visiting native villages, especially at night.

The use of DDT powder, sprinkled in the seams of garments (for lice and fleas), in beds and cracks where insects collect (for fleas, roaches, bedbugs and ticks).

CLASS III

EXTRA PRECAUTIONS AGAINST CERTAIN DISEASES

(See lists of diseases, pages 271–273)

1. Refraining from wading or bathing in untreated fresh water or in salt water contaminated by fresh-water streams or by sewage.
2. Refraining from walking barefoot on the soil or handling soil without the use of gloves.
3. Refraining from touching people or animals with sores.
4. Refraining from intimacy with dogs employed in caring for sheep.
5. Use of a bed net with an extra-fine mesh or applying repellent to bed mat (page 156).

6. Refraining from sleeping on the floor.
7. Measures against ticks (page 159).
8. Immunization.
9. The use of certain drugs for suppression or prophylaxis:
   (*a*) Aralen for suppression of malaria (page 264). This is only for regions of high endemicity, as shown on the map.
   (*b*) Tablets of milibis and aralen combined, for prevention of amoebic dysentery. To be used only when danger is acute, as when ordinary precautions cannot be taken, and only for periods of not more than 3 months. Tablets of diodoquin, used for 20 days, are an alternative for prevention of amoebic dysentery.
   (*c*) Sulfadiazine tablets for prevention of bacillary dysentery. To be used only when danger is acute, as at time of an epidemic.
   (*d*) Stovarsol (acetarsone) tablets for prevention of relapsing fever, conveyed by ticks in central Africa, sometimes called "African tick fever" (used in preparation for journeys through infected regions).
   (*e*) One intramuscular injection of pentamidine will protect against trypanosomiasis (African sleeping sickness) for 6 months (used in preparation for journeys through infected regions).

INDEX

▬▬

NOTE: Italic page numbers, when used, refer to the main discussion of an item.